PREPARATION FOR
MRCP Part II

PREPARATION FOR MRCP Part II

Paul Siklos and
Stephen Olczak

Published, in association with
UPDATE PUBLICATIONS LTD., by

1983 **MTP PRESS LIMITED**
a member of the KLUWER ACADEMIC PUBLISHERS GROUP
BOSTON / THE HAGUE / DORDRECHT / LANCASTER

Published in the UK and Europe,
in association with Update Publications Ltd., by
MTP Press Limited
Falcon House
Lancaster, England

British Library Cataloguing in Publication Data

Siklos, Paul
    Preparation for MRCP Part II.
    1. Medicine—Problems, exercises, etc.
    I. Title   II. Olczak, Stephen
    610'.76   P834.5

    ISBN-13: 978-94-011-7303-2   e-ISBN-13: 978-94-011-7301-8
    DOI: 10.1007/978-94-011-7301-8

Published in the USA by
MTP Press
A division of Kluwer Boston Inc
190 Old Derby Street
Hingham, MA 02043, USA

Library of Congress Cataloging in Publication Data

Siklos, Paul.
    Preparation for MRCP part II.

    Includes index.
    1. Internal medicine-Examinations, questions, etc.
I. Olczak, Stephen.   II. Title.   III. Title: Preparation for M.R.C.P.
part II.   IV. Title: Preparation for MRCP part 2.   [DNLM: 1.
Medicine-Examination questions. W 18 S579p]
RC58.S54 1983   616'.0076   83-13213
ISBN-13: 978-94-011-7303-2

Copyright © 1983 Paul Siklos and Stephen Olczak
Softcover reprint of the hardcover 1st edition 1983

Reprinted 1985

CONTENTS

THE AUTHORS

Paul Siklos, MA, BSc, MB, MRCP
Consultant Physician, West Suffolk Hospital, Bury St Edmunds and
Newmarket General Hospital;
Recognized Clinical Teacher, University of Cambridge, UK

Stephen Olczak, BSc, MD, MRCP
Honorary Senior Registrar in Medicine, Addenbrooke's Hospital,
Cambridge, UK

PREFACE

This book is directed towards post-graduates who have passed Part I of the examination for Membership of the Royal College of Physicians and are preparing for Part II. However, it is hoped that physicians at all stages of their careers will find some parts that interest them. Most of the material has appeared in the *Hospital Update* series, 'Preparation for MRCP', but this has been modified and expanded; many useful points arising from correspondence relating to the series have been included, and the authors would like to express their thanks to those who have written. It is not intended that this should be used as a work of reference, although there is detailed discussion of some subjects.

Only the written part of the examination is dealt with in detail, but the introduction contains hints on tackling the clinical sections which the authors hope the candidates will find valuable. There is, however, no substitute for clinical practice under supervision. The questions in the written section of the examination require short answers so that marking may be easy and objective. This book contains questions similar to those that may be encountered in the examination, but the answers have been expanded as a basis for discussion. It is hoped that this will encourage the candidate to read around the subjects covered, and the authors recommend that the questions are used as a basis for group discussion, as answers other than those in the text may be considered.

There are sections dealing with case histories; data for interpretation (including advice on interpretation of cardiac catheter data); colour slides of clinical material and slides of radiographs with examination-orientated hints on interpretation of the radiographs of the chest, abdomen and skull.

The authors gratefully acknowledge contributions from: Dr Nick Boon; Mr Neil Rushton; Dr Carol Seymour; Dr David Stone; Dr Richard Greenwood; and Dr Geoff Tobin, as co-author of the first 8 articles in the Update series. We would also like to thank Dr David Rubenstein for his help and advice in the preparation of the articles for *Hospital Update*. The authors are particularly grateful to Dr Ray Godwin for advice about the radiographs presented, and for the hints on interpretation of X-rays of the chest, abdomen and skull.

The authors would also like to thank Samantha Loftus and Lesley Stellitano for typing the manuscript, and Marcia Thorburn for the line drawings.

Finally, they would like to express their thanks to Mr Phil Johnstone of MTP Press Ltd for his encouragement and patience.

January, 1983

INTRODUCTION

The MRCP (UK) examination is an entrance examination designed to select those who are suitable for higher specialist training in general internal medicine and its related specialities. The achievement of this diploma is essential in order to progress to higher training and a career in hospital medicine. Those who pass the examination will have a firm basic knowledge of medicine; will be able to take a history, and examine a patient in a professional and accurate manner; and will be able to plan a rational course of management for patients presenting with common problems. Many successful candidates have commented that the examination is similar to the MB Final examination but that mistakes are more heavily penalized and a greater degree of professionalism is required.

The examination is divided into 2 parts. Part I was introduced in 1968 as a screening examination, because prior to this each candidate

1

had a clinical bedside test and as the number taking the examination increased there was a considerable strain on resources. The Part I examination consists of 60 multiple choice questions, and in addition to filtering out those candidates suitable for progressing to Part II it is the only part of the examination to test a wide range of factual knowledge. It has been shown that those who pass Part I by a narrow margin perform less well at Part II than those who passed the Part I examination more convincingly.

The candidate is not eligible to enter for Part II of the examination until he has completed a period of at least 30 months of approved clinical experience following graduation. Of this 18 months is post-registration experience, and 12 of these months must be spent in posts that include the emergency care of patients (either children or adults) acutely ill with general medical conditions. Rather than inspect and approve each training post the College requires that a candidate who presents himself for Part II should produce two testimonials from Fellows of the Colleges or from Members of 8 years standing. The sponsors testify that the candidate has the necessary experience and suitable character, and that he is ready to take Part II.

The Part II examination is divided into two parts, the written and the clinical separated by about a month. The candidate must pass the written section of the examination before proceeding to the clinical part, but the pass may be so borderline that bonus marks from the clinical examination will be required in order to produce a pass for the whole of Part II.

WRITTEN SECTION

Factual medical knowledge has been tested in Part I of the examination and this part asks the candidate to solve clinical problems, to interpret data and to comment on projected material (radiographs and clinical photographs). Written essays were abandoned because of the unrelia-bility of the marking due to examiner variability, the limited range of subject matter which can be tested and the demands made on the examiners' time. The questions are produced by examiners and sub-mitted to a Board in London. Some are selected and refined, and then passed to the Colleges in Edinburgh and Glasgow where they are further criticized before being put into the bank. The questions are often refined still further before being used. The questions generate answers (as opposed to multiple choice questions) and the questions are designed so that the answers should be short, objective and easily corrected. Acceptable answers with appropriate marks have been drawn up and irrelevant answers receive no marks. A penalty may be incurred for suggestions which are likely to be harmful to the patient.

Case Histories (Grey Cases)

There are 4 or more compulsory questions to be discussed in 55 minutes. Each states the history, physical signs and results of investigations. The questions are phrased so as to elicit brief answers that can be marked objectively. Typical questions would be 'List 3 probable diagnoses', 'Suggest 4 investigations which would be helpful in the diagnosis'. Maximum marks would be awarded to answers which have been agreed by the Board as being the best response. All answers contain potentially the same number of marks, and it seems, therefore, reasonable to suggest a sensible answer that you are not sure about rather than to leave a question unanswered.

Some of the information given in the Case will be irrelevant but none should be actually misleading. It is often useful to concentrate on aspects of the Case for which there is an established list of causes (e.g. the presence of clubbing, haemoptysis, etc). Any diagnosis must take account of these. Remember that rare presentations of common diseases are commoner than the common presentation of a rare disease, and in general it is your ability to deal with common diseases that is being tested.

Data Interpretation

There are 10 sets of data to be interpreted in 45 minutes. The material includes biochemical, endocrinological and haematological profiles, electrocardiograms, lung function studies, cardiac catherization data, analysis of urine and cerebro-spinal fluid, all usually preceded by a brief clinical abstract. The questions again call for brief, objective answers and the preferred answer receives maximum marks. You must be fully conversant with the normal ranges of values for commonly used investigations.

Projected Material

A slide (or pair of slides) is shown for 90 seconds. A bell then rings and a further 30 seconds is allowed before the slide changes. Candidates are asked to answer brief questions on each slide by writing on the combined question and answer sheet provided. There may be a brief history accompanying the slide and questions may be asked about the documentation of abnormalities shown, likely diagnosis or differential diagnosis, likely presenting symptoms etc. There are 20 slides, about a quarter of which are radiographs, and these may include arteriograms, myelograms or barium studies. There is usually a peripheral blood film or bone marrow aspirate and a histology slide. Seating in the lecture theatre is arranged so that each candidate has a good view of the screen and the pictures are of a high standard. A picture of an optic fundus would be preceded by a normal picture to demonstrate photographic artefacts. It is worth being familiar with the appearance of common dermatological conditions.

CLINICAL SECTION

Those who pass the written examination proceed to the *viva*, and to the short and long cases. Approximately a quarter of those taking the written Part of the exam will fail but the failure rate of the clinical Part is not disclosed. It is likely, however, that the failure rate is high, and this may be because candidates have insufficient competence, knowledge or experience. However, many fail because of poor presentation and lack of technique. These are areas that can be considerably improved by practice. When face to face with the examiner the following general points are worth considering.

(1) Appearance is very important.
   During the clinical section you will meet 3 pairs of examiners and first impressions are vital. Dress should be conservative, and club and old school ties avoided. Smell should be neutral.
(2) Try to relax and impress the examiner with your quiet confident ability.
   This implies that you function well in stressful situations, and will make a good hospital doctor. A candidate may possibly fail because the examiners feel that he is just not suitable to be a consultant physician and Member of the College despite otherwise adequate performance.
(3) However, do not be over-confident and dogmatic particularly when discussing controversial issues.
   You are being tested on general clinical medicine, and not on the latest breakthrough in an obscure sub-speciality with which you happen to be conversant.

(4) Never argue with the examiners even though you 'know' that you are correct.

(5) You should demonstrate that you know the commonest causes of conditions.

However, if you are confident you can start with a rare but *treatable* cause which is not to be missed. Always try and talk from general to specific and from common to rare.

(6) Avoid abbreviations.

A string of apparently unconnected letters is annoying and confusing and may also be misleading e.g. MI may be mitral incompetence or myocardial infarction, PID – pelvic inflammatory disease or prolapsed intervertebral disc and RIF may mean right iliac fossa or right index finger.

Oral examination

This is often the first confrontation between examiners and examinee, and is often very informative for the former and nerve-wracking for the latter. There are 2 examiners who each conduct an interview of approximately 10 minutes (20 minutes in total). At least 3 or 4 topics are covered and each examiner marks all the time, and at the end of the 20 minutes each writes down his mark before further discussion. Because factual knowledge has been fully assessed in previous sections the *viva* concentrates mainly on testing the candidate on the management of medical emergencies, basic scientific principles and the ability to deal with specific clinical situations. An increasing emphasis is being placed on sociological and psychological aspects of patient care, and the examiner may take the opportunity of asking your opinion on topical aspects of medical ethics. The candidate may sometimes be asked to complete a form saying where he is working and what job he is doing. The first question may then relate to the appropriate speciality or unit. A question to an SHO in Neurology may be 'Discuss the appliances available to help the rehabilitation of a stroke patient' rather than a request for neurological facts. Topical problems include drug addiction, alcoholism, patient compliance and problems of the elderly. It is useful to read the leading articles of the *British Medical Journal*, *Lancet* and *New England Journal of Medicine* for a few months before the *viva*.

Ensure that you arrive early enough to be fully composed by the time you are called in. First impressions are important, and if it is obvious that you are disorganized enough to be late for the interview the

5

examiners will conclude that your attitude to medicine is equally disorganized. You will also lack the confidence required to be seen at your best. A neatly dressed candidate who looks alert, intelligent and enthusiastic will have an immediate advantage over someone who is slovenly and lethargic. Take the proffered chair politely, and exchange any pleasantries which may be offered. The first question is usually straightforward and gives time to develop rapport. Consider the following points:

(1) Do not repeat the question while thinking of an answer. This is a most irritating habit.

(2) Try and plan your answer so that the most important aspects are mentioned first, particularly if the question is voiced in general terms. For example, in reply to the question 'Discuss the treatment of thyrotoxicosis' it is important to start 'There are 3 choices – anti-thyroid drugs, radio-iodine and surgery' and then discuss each in more depth.

(3) In the event of not understanding a question say you are not clear exactly what is being asked and the examiner will re-phrase the question. If you ask him to repeat the question he may well do so and you will be no further forward. In addition you will have wasted time and probably irritated the examiner.

(4) You must admit early on that you know nothing about the subject under discussion if this is the case. This will eventually be deduced and valuable time which could be used discussing a more familiar subject will be lost. However, it is important that you do not 'pass' on too many questions!

(5) Be prepared to discuss a pathological specimen or radiograph. It is usually wise to describe the exhibit as accurately as possible before further discussion.

(6) Try and concentrate on what you are saying and avoid vague and meaningless phrases. Your ability to communicate as well as your medical knowledge and judgement is being assessed.

(7) It pays to keep the discussion as simple as possible unless you are very sure of the subject. The mention of rare eponymous syndromes (of which the examiner may well not have heard) often causes antagonism.

At the end of the allotted time leave graciously after thanking the examiners. Such an exit leaves a good impression and may sway judgement in borderline circumstances.

Short Cases

You are now introduced to a different pair of examiners and asked to demonstrate your skill in eliciting and interpreting physical signs. The examiners have no knowledge of your previous performance and again an initial good impression is vital. The total time allotted to the short cases has been increased from 20 to 30 minutes because the examiners feel that this is one of the best areas to assess clinical skills. It is the section that candidates fear most, and there is no substitute for practice. The examiners hope to cover 4 out of the 5 major systems and also show 2 or 3 'spot cases'. Each examiner marks all the time independently, and marks are written down at the end before conferring.

The examiners are assessing your technique so a certain amount of showmanship is called for. Be methodical, accurate and comprehensive and make sure the examiner knows what you are doing. Make a point of inspection because although you may have noticed the signs to be seen on inspection, it is important that you are seen doing so. Every action should be clear and simple and look well practised. You must make up your mind about a sign on first (or at worst) second examination, as there is nothing worse than having to watch repeated half-hearted demonstrations of physical signs. A sign is either abnormal or it is not - avoid words such as minimal, slight, minor, a hint of cyanosis, clubbing etc. Never say that you searched for a physical sign but could not elicit it. It would be incompetent to miss palpating an enlarged spleen, but to suggest that you examined carefully and still missed it makes matters worse. Some candidates find that giving a running commentary of findings saves time but others prefer to sum up at the end. If you feel confident you may state a diagnosis, otherwise summarize the positive findings.

It is well known that some examiners tend to be aggressive (the hawks) and some benign (the doves). Hawks and doves are often paired together, and candidates often try to direct attention towards the dove who appears more sympathetic. However, remember that both examiners are marking all the time. The examiner will often introduce the patient by name and will provide a short case history. He will then give instructions as to what he wishes you to do. These instructions are brief and should be explicit but it is important to understand what is required so ask for clarification if there is any doubt. Examination of the 'heart' is different to 'the cardiovascular system' but if asked to do the former it is worth commenting, for the sake of completeness, that

Table Possible short cases: a list based on candidates' recent experiences

Cardiovascular
Common congenital heart disease (ASD, VSD etc.)
Valvular disease of the heart
Prosthetic valves
Coarctation of the aorta
Hypertrophic cardiomyopathy
Jugular venous pressure

Respiratory
Chronic obstructive disease
Clubbing
Fibrosing alveolitis

Gastrointestinal
Hepatomegaly
Splenomegaly
Ascites
Chronic liver failure
Tongue
Primary biliary cirrhosis

Haematology
Lymphadenopathy
Purpuric rash

Fundoscopy (see Hurst, G. (1979). Examination of the eye. *Hospital Update*, 1979, 5, 1137)
Diabetes
Hypertension
Optic atrophy, papilloedema
Retinal artery/vein occlusion
Cataract

Endocrine
Thyroid swelling, hypo- and hyperthyroidism
Acromegaly
Gynaecomastia
Diabetic complications
Cushing's syndrome
Turner's syndrome

Neurology
Chronic neurological syndromes:
    Multiple sclerosis
    Dystrophia myotonica
    Motor neurone disease
    Syringomyelia
    Parkinsonian syndrome
    Tabes dorsalis
    Friedreich's ataxia
    Muscular dystrophies

Visual field abnormalities
Nystagmus
Pupillary abnormalities
Horner's syndrome
Diplopia

Cranial nerve palsies (III, IV, VI, VII)
Cerebellar syndromes
Bulbar/pseudobulbar palsies
Dysarthria
Hydrocephalus

Gait disorders
Peripheral neuropathy
Peripheral nerve injuries
Wasting of the small muscles of the hand

Musculoskeletal
Osteoarthrosis
Gout
Rheumatoid disease – arthritis and systemic manifestations
Scoliosis
Ankylosing spondylitis
Collagen disease:
    Scleroderma, CREST syndrome
    SLE
    Dermatomyositis
Marfan's syndrome
Neurofibromatosis

Table (continued)

Dermatology	Nephrological
Common skin lesions and those associated with systemic disease	Neuropathic bladder Uraemia, shunts, fistulae Polycystic kidneys

you would look at the hands, ankles and so on but spend time only on the heart itself. Similarly, it is worth trying to get as much information from other systems as possible but time should not be wasted on doing other than the examiners ask. You should try and greet the patient by his name (if told) and ask permission to examine the part concerned. The examiner may then say 'of course he does not mind you examining him, that is why he is here'. However, it is important to approach patients with respect and treat them as fellow humans rather than as objects to be examined. The candidate may have elicited all the signs correctly but still fail because of a rude or callous approach to the patient. Remember to use euphemisms for diseases such as cancer, syphilis or epilepsy when talking within earshot of a patient. Do not ask the patients any leading questions which may help in the diagnosis as this is supposed to be achieved by physical examination alone.

It is very useful when preparing for the examination to make a list of possible short cases and to write down the physical signs which may be associated with each condition (see the Table). Plan a methodical approach to each problem, e.g. if you are shown a patient with acromegaly and asked to demonstrate evidence of any complications you should be able quickly to assess visual fields, look for median nerve compression and so on. It is particularly useful to rehearse patient examination and presentation in the presence of a critical audience (your Consultant or Senior Registrar). This will ensure that your method of examination is not only correct, logical and thorough but also that it is carried out with style and professionalism.

Long Case

You are given access to a patient for 60 minutes and are required to take a full history, make a clinical examination and perform any bedside or side-room tests (such as urinalysis) which you consider appropriate. At the end of that time you will meet a further pair of examiners one of whom does most of the examining, but again each marks individually and they confer at the end. The examiners will require an accurate, concise history; a brief synopsis of the physical signs (which you may be asked to demonstrate) and a presentation of the problems of diagnosis, further investigation and management. The examiners will be interested in a presentation of the patient's problems, not only physical but also mental and social.

The patients chosen for the examination tend to be new Out-patients and In-patients rather than the 'MRCP exam chronic cases', who are practised at churning out their 'classical' (but rare) history and demonstrating a bewildering array of physical signs. A working diagnosis has usually been reached and the patients often present more than one problem. There may be very few physical signs, and the aim of the long case is to assess technique of history taking and presentation and solution of patients' problems. For these reasons traditional examination shortcuts such as the opening gambit 'What do the doctors say is wrong with you?' are less relevant. Approach the patient as you would a new case in the clinic rather than change your routine to attempt to play 'the long case game'. However, when you have completed your assessment and formed your own impression, it is worth asking the patient if he knows his diagnosis and what investigations he has had done.

It is very important to ensure that you have at least 10 minutes for thought before meeting the examiners. During this time the main points can be mentally rehearsed, because this is the only situation where you have a chance to run the interview, by steering the conversation towards subjects about which you are familiar. It is important to take a problem orientated approach and say how the illness affects the patient. You must anticipate any questions about differential diagnosis, further investigations and future management of the patient. It is very important to make your presentation interesting.

General Points

The clinical section tests command of clinical skills and enables the examiner to assess your attitude towards patients. It is very important to have practice in talking to and examining patients with as wide a variety of diseases as possible. A busy general medical job is ideal for this. It soon becomes obvious when a candidate is at ease with patients and can confidentially elicit physical signs, and this approach comes automatically to those with a wide range of clinical experience. Be sure that you can wield a patella hammer and use an ophthalmoscope. It is often worth taking your own equipment to the examination as you will be familiar with it, and will not have to compete with other harassed candidates for ward items. It is certainly worth having in your possession a hat pin for testing visual fields, an orange stick for eliciting the plantar response and a tape measure.

It is difficult to plan specific reading for the clinical part of the examination as the field is so extensive. There is no substitute for seeing patients in a clinical setting and presenting such patients to a critical audience. However, many candidates have found the following of considerable help:

1. Beck, E. R. Francis, J. L. and Souhami, R. L. (1982). *Tutorials in Differential Diagnosis*. 2nd edn. (Edinburgh: Churchill Livingstone)
2. Mason, S. and Swash, M. (1980). *Hutchison's Clinical Methods*. 17th edn. (London: Baillière-Tindall)
3. Ogilvie, C. (1980). *Chamberlain's Symptoms and Signs in Clinical Medicine: an Introduction to Medical Diagnosis*. 10th edn. (Bristol: Wright)
4. Pappworth, M. H. (1985). *Primer of Medicine*. 5th edn. (Sevenoaks: Butterworths)
5. Rubenstein, D. and Wayne, D. (1985). *Lecture Notes on Clinical Medicine*. 3rd edn. (Oxford: Blackwell Scientific)
6. Zatouroff, M. (1976). *A Colour Atlas of Physical Signs in General Medicine*. Wolfe Medical Atlases, No. 16. (London: Wolfe)

The following papers relating to the examination and examination technique are also useful:

1. Cohen, J. A. (1982). Postgraduate Diplomas MRCP Part II. *Br. J. Hosp. Med.*, **28**, 361
2. Constable, T. J. (1975). A guide to preparing for the MRCP (UK) exam. *Hospital Update*, 635
3. Shinton, N. K. (1978). How to take an examination viva. *Br. Med. J.*, **2**, 1694
4. Smith, R. (1982). Becoming a member of the Royal College of Physicians; trial by MCQ. *Br. Med. J.*, **2**, 1341
5. Stokes, J. F. (1979). How to take a clinical examination. *Br. Med. J.*, **1**: 98
6. Symposium MRCP: 1977 (1978). *Br. Med. J.*, **1**, 217.

TABLE OF NORMAL VALUES

(approximate SI conversion to conventional units is given in brackets)

Haematology

(note g/dl = mg/100 ml and $1 \times 10^9/l = 1000$ cells/mm³)

Haemoglobin (Hb) Male   13.5-17.5 g/dl
                 Female 12.5-16.5 g/dl
Packed cell volume (PCV) 0.40-0.54 l/l
Mean cell volume (MCV) 77-93 fl
Mean cell haemoglobin concentration (MCHC) 29-35 g/dl
Reticulocytes 0.2-2.0% ($10-100 \times 10^9/l$)
Leucocyte count (WCC) $4.0-11.0 \times 10^9/l$
Differential leucocyte count: Neutrophils $2.0-7.5 \times 10^9/l$ (40-75%)
                                 Lymphocytes $1.5-4.0 \times 10^9/l$ (20-45%)
                                 Monocytes $0.2-0.8 \times 10^9/l$ (2-10%)
                                 Eosinophils $0.04-0.4 \times 10^9/l$ (1-6%)
                                 Basophils $<0.01-0.1 \times 10^9/l$ (1%)
Platelet count $150-400 \times 10^9/l$
Serum $B_{12} > 130$ ng/l
Serum folate 3-13 μg/l
Red cell folate > 150 μg/l

Plasma Urea and Electrolytes

Sodium	132-142	mmol/l (= mEq/l)
Potassium	3.4-5.0	mmol/l (= mEq/l)
Bicarbonate	22-30	mmol/l (= mEq/l)
Glucose	3.5-9.0	mmol/l ($\times 18 =$ mg/dl)
Urea	up to 7.5	mmol/l ($\times 6 =$ mg/dl)
Creatinine	35-125	μmol/l ($\times 0.011 =$ mg/dl)

Liver and Bone Tests

Total protein	63-83	g/l ($\div 10 =$ g/dl)
Albumin	30-44	g/l
Calcium	2.20-2.60	mmol/l ($\times 4 =$ mg/dl)
Phosphate	0.80-1.40	mmol/l ($\times 3 =$ mg/dl)
Bilirubin (Total)	up to 17	μmol/l ($\times 0.058 =$ mg/dl)
Alkaline phosphatase	30-135	U/l
SGPT (ALT)	7-40	U/l

Urinary Urea and Electrolytes

Sodium	50-200 mmol/24 h
Potassium	20-60 mmol/24 h
Urea	330-500 mmol/24 h
Creatinine	9.0-16 mmol/24 h
Creatinine clearance	90-110 ml/min
Calcium	2.8-7.5 mmol/24 h
Phosphate	22-32 mmol/24 h

Serum Protein Electrophoresis

Transferrin	2.2-3.8 g/l
IgG	6.0-13.0 g/l
IgA	0.8-3.7 g/l
IgM	0.4-2.2 g/l
Alpha-1-antitrypsin	0.9-1.8 g/l
Haptoglobin	0.5-2.6 g/l

Arterial Blood Gases

Hydrogen ion	36-45 nmol/l
pH	7.35-7.45
P_{O_2}	9.3-13.3 kPa ($\times 7.5 = $ mmHg)
P_{CO_2}	4.6-6.0 kPa

Miscellaneous Biochemistry

Acid phosphatase		up to 0.7 U/l
Cortisol		280-650 nmol/l ($\times 0.036 = \mu g/dl$)
Creatine kinase	Male	24-195 U/l
	Female	24-170 U/l
Growth hormone, fasting		< 10 mU/l
Insulin, fasting		< 25 mU/l
Iron	Male	14-32 μmol/l ($\times 5.6 = \mu g/dl$)
	Female	10-28 μmol/l
Prolactin	Male	< 150 mU/l
	Female	< 300 mU/l
SGOT		< 35 U/l
Thyroxine (total T4)		65-145 nmol/l (4-12 $\mu g/dl$)
Triiodothyronine (Total T3)		1.0-2.8 nmol/l
TSH		< 4.0 mU/l
Uric acid		0.12-0.45 mmol/l ($\times 17 = $ mg/dl)

Cerebrospinal Fluid

Protein	0.1–0.4 g/l
Glucose	>70% of simultaneous blood glucose
Cells – Lymphocytes	<3/mm³

Section 1
CASE HISTORIES

Q1 A 15-year-old girl presents as an emergency with a 12-hour history of fever, confusion, diarrhoea and vomiting. Her parents when questioned say that for the previous two months she has complained of diarrhoea with no blood or mucus and has lost weight in spite of a good appetite. Her mother has insulin-dependent diabetes.

On examination, she is confused and agitated with no skin rash. Other observations are: temperature 40°C; pulse 140 per minute, irregular; blood pressure 90/60 mmHg; abdomen normal; rectal examination normal, soft faeces.

Investigations show:
Haemoglobin 15 g/dl
White cell count $16 \times 10^9/l$
Platelets $400 \times 10^9/l$
Sodium 143 mmol/l, potassium 3.2 mmol/l, urea 18 mmol/l, creatinine 140 μmol/l
Plasma glucose 6.5 mmol/l
Calcium 2.92 mmol/l, phosphate 1.9 mmol/l, albumin 43 g/l

Questions:
(1) What is the most likely diagnosis?
(2) What urgent investigations would you request?
(3) Outline your management of this condition.

Q2 A 16-year-old girl, who one week previously returned from a holiday in southern Spain is admitted with a 2-day history of watery diarrhoea, fever, vomiting and headache. She had had unprotected sexual intercourse while abroad, but had been menstruating normally for the 3 days prior to admission. The other members of the party had not had similar symptoms.

She is confused with a temperature of 40°C, flushed and toxic, with bilateral conjunctivitis. Her skin shows a diffuse erythematous macular rash resembling sunburn. Her blood pressure is 80 mmHg systolic with a pulse rate of 130 per minute. There is no clinical evidence of pneumonia.

Investigations show:
Hb 13.5 g/dl

White cell count $17 \times 10^9/l$ (90% neutrophils)
Platelets $40 \times 10^9/l$
Plasma sodium 129 mmol/l, potassium 3.2 mmol/l, urea 15 mmol/l, creatinine 220 μmol/l, glucose 6 mmol/l
Lumbar puncture shows clear fluid containing 3 red cells and 2 lymphocytes. CSF glucose is 4 mmol/l
Cultures of blood and stool on 4 occasions are negative. A high vaginal swab grew staphylococcus aureus. Monospot test is negative and a chest radiograph normal.

Questions:
(1) What is the likely diagnosis?
(2) What would be your initial and long-term management?

A 55-year-old woman with well controlled insulin-dependent diabetes of 10 years' duration presents with a history of postural dizziness. She denies palpitation. She suffered from a myocardial infarction complicated by left ventricular failure 6 months previously, and since then has been taking frusemide 40 mg and amiloride 10 mg each twice daily.

Q3

Her pulse is 110 per minute regular. Supine blood pressure is 135/90 mmHg and standing blood pressure 95/70 mmHg. There is bilateral background retinopathy and deep tendon reflexes at the ankles are absent. Examination is otherwise normal.

Investigations show:
Plasma sodium 120 mmol/l, potassium 3.3 mmol/l, bicarbonate 29 mmol/l, urea 14.5 mmol/l, creatinine 125 μmol/l; glucose 12.9 mmol/l.

Questions:
(1) Suggest 2 possible mechanisms to explain her symptoms.
(2) How would you investigate these?
(3) What treatment might you suggest for each?

Q4

A 61-year-old man with no significant past medical history developed an influenza-like illness associated with low back pain of moderate severity. His systemic symptoms cleared after 48 hours but he was left with back pain and diffuse muscle pains in both legs. Five days later he complains of increasing difficulty in walking because of the leg weakness and is admitted to hospital where he develops urinary retention.

He is alert and orientated with minimal neck stiffness and a temperature of 38°C. He is tender over the lower lumbar spine with reduction of straight leg raising to 30° bilaterally because of back pain. The lower extremeties are flaccid, and distal weakness in the arms is noted. Sensation is normal except for diminished appreciation to pinprick over the dorsum and sole of the right foot. Deep tendon reflexes at the knees and ankles are absent. No plantar responses are elicited and anal sphincter tone is diminished. Examination is otherwise normal.

Investigations are:

Chest radiograph normal

Lumbar spine radiograph shows narrowing of L4/5 disc space

Cerebro-spinal fluid:

    red cells 25 000 /mm³

    lymphocytes 10/mm³

    neutrophils 30/mm³

    glucose 5 mmol/l (simultaneous blood glucose 7 mmol/l)

    protein 2.8 g/l

Questions:

(1) What is the most likely diagnosis?

(2) Give 2 differential diagnoses

(3) Explain why the 2 conditions in Question 2 are less likely than the condition chosen as the most likely diagnosis.

Q5

A 27-year-old unmarried nurse presents with a 3 month history of episodes of faintness, dizziness and palpitation, usually occurring shortly after rising in the morning. These episodes were becoming more frequent. On 2 occasions she had experienced similar symptoms following a long game of tennis in the late morning but had recently stopped playing because of weight gain. Five years previously she had been admitted overnight following an episode of self-poisoning with benzodiazepines. Reactive depression, following the break-up of an affair with a married man, was diagnosed by the psychiatrist who saw her. For several months she had been behaving rather oddly at home and at work, and nursing colleagues had been putting pressure on her to re-establish contact with the psychiatrist.

A younger sister has insulin-dependent diabetes mellitus. There is no other relevant previous medical history or family history.

Apart from generalized obesity, physical examination is entirely normal.

Questions:
(1) Describe how you would investigate such a patient.
(2) What is the most likely diagnosis?

A 25-year-old patient with Down's Syndrome presents with breathlessness and is found to be anaemic. He is taking phenytoin for long-standing epilepsy which has been well controlled and he denies any other drug ingestion.

Q6

For a few years previously he has had episodes of back pain and dark urine. Three months prior to being seen his mother (with whom he lives) noted he was off his food and had become jaundiced (again with dark urine) but he recovered after 2 weeks with no medical intervention.

Investigations show:
Haemoglobin 5 g/dl
MCV 105 fl
White cell count 1.7×10^9/l
Film shows a normal distribution of cells with no abnormal cells
Platelets 40×10^9/l

Questions:
(1) Give 4 possible causes for the haematological abnormalities.
(2) What would be the single most useful investigation?

Q7

A 68-year-old man presents with bilateral pitting leg oedema with no elevation of the jugular venous pressure. He has 10 cm hepatomegaly which is smooth and firm. The spleen is not palpable and there is no ascites.

Investigations show:

Haemoglobin 13.3 g/dl

White cell count 8.2 × 10⁹/l (normal differential)

ESR 115 mm/first h

Clotting screen normal

Plasma, electrolytes, urea and creatinine normal

Albumin 24 g/l, alkaline phosphatase 750 U/l, SGPT and bilirubin normal

Protein electrophoresis shows IgG M-band with immune paresis

24 h urinary protein excretion 12.5 g (Bence Jones protein negative)

Electrocardiogram normal, but of low voltage

⁹⁹Tc pyrophosphate bone scan normal

Questions:

(1) Give 3 possible diagnoses.

(2) Give 5 useful investigations to assist in establishing a diagnosis.

Q8

A 71-year-old woman living in the South of France is admitted comatose with a 1 year history of episodes of confusion. Diabetes mellitus had been diagnosed 10 years previously, and had been treated initially with oral hypoglycaemic agents but more recently has been well controlled by insulin. Her only other medication is indomethacin for arthritis of the knees, but until 2 months previously she had been taking a tricyclic antidepressant. Her husband said that she usually drank a bottle of wine with her evening meal and that she did not smoke. Her level of consciousness had been deteriorating for several days and he noted that she was sleeping during the day and roaming about the house at night.

Examination shows her to be suntanned and responding only to painful stimuli. The pulse is 90/minute, blood pressure 110/70. The tendon reflexes are increased and the plantar responses extensor but there are no other neurological signs.

Initial investigations show:
  Blood glucose 7.0 mmol/l
  Plasma sodium 127 mmol/l, potassium 3.9 mmol/l, urea 1.4 mmol/l
  Lumbar puncture: CSF pressure 120 mm H_2O, 15 red cells/mm³,
  2 lymphocytes/mm³, protein 0.4 g/l, glucose 5 mmol/l

Questions:
(1) What is the likely cause of her coma?
(2) Give 3 causes for the underlying pathology.
(3) Give 4 helpful investigations.

Q9

A 56-year-old psychiatric nurse presents with weakness and diarrhoea. He gives a 3 month history of dry cough, and during this time has lost 7 kg in weight. He admits to recent nocturia and polyuria. He is a heavy cigarette smoker and he and his wife own a sweet and cigarette shop which she manages. Ten years previously he was investigated for episodic abdominal pain, and a barium meal then showed scarring of the duodenum. Since then he has experienced recurrent epigastric pain for which he takes self-prescribed medication. There is a 5-year history of hypertension and again the drug therapy is managed by the patient himself.

Examination shows an unwell man, clinically dehydrated. Apart from a blood pressure of 170/110 mmHg and tenderness in the epigastrium there are no other abnormal physical signs.

Initial investigations show:
  A normal blood count
  Plasma sodium 139 mmol/l, potassium 2.3 mmol/l, bicarbonate
  34 mmol/l, urea 9 mmol/l, creatinine 120 μmol/l,
  glucose 7 mmol/l

Questions:
(1) Give 4 possible causes to account for these results.
(2) Give 3 possible causes for his polyuria.

21

Q10 A 72-year-old man is admitted with a 1 month history of right-sided pleuritic chest pain, a dry cough and 4 kilogram weight loss. He has had no haemoptysis but for several years has noticed progressive breathlessness. For 20 years he worked in a shipyard and he retired at the age of 60. He smokes 20 cigarettes a day.

Examination shows an ill man with a respiratory rate of 40/minute, temperature 37°C and digital clubbing. No lymph nodes are palpable. There is dullness to percussion and diminished breath sounds over the lower half of the right lung.

Initial investigations are:

Haemoglobin 14.1 g/dl

White cell count $5.4 \times 10^9/l$ (65% neutrophils)

Chest radiograph shows a normal left lung and a right pleural effusion.

Pleural aspiration is performed and 900 ml of fluid is obtained.

Analysis of this shows:

Red blood cells 700/mm³

White cells 9000/mm³   50% mesothelial cells

                                             35% lymphocytes

                                             15% polymorphs

Culture shows no growth.

A repeat chest radiograph (PA and lateral) shows pleural thickening but no parenchymal lung lesion. 3 days later a further chest radiograph shows that the fluid has reaccumulated.

Questions:

(1) What investigation would you perform next?

(2) Suggest 2 likely diagnoses.

Q11 A previously well 50-year-old woman with a normal diet and taking no medication presents with a painless swelling of the thyroid gland of 3 months' duration. There is no significant family history.

She is clinically euthyroid and has no dysthyroid eye disease. She has an irregular, firm, mobile goitre with the left lobe markedly enlarged but the isthmus and right lobe can still be determined. No regional lymph nodes are palpable.

Investigations show:
serum thyroxine 50 nmol/l, TSH 22 mU/l
serum calcium 2.8 mmol/l, phosphate 0.9 mmol/l, albumin 40 g/l,
alkaline phosphatase 90 U/l.

Questions:
(1) Give 3 possible diagnoses.
(2) Give 3 investigations which would aid diagnosis.
(3) What would be the management of each of the 3 diagnoses when
applied to the above patient?

A 62-year-old Greek Cypriot woman with severe rheumatoid arthritis
presents with a 2 month history of breathlessness on exertion, gradually
increasing ankle oedema and generalized pruritus. She has a long
history of well controlled hypertension, but is unsure of the drugs she
is taking.

Q12

Examination shows an over-weight, slightly icteric and anaemic lady
with oedema to the thighs, who is apyrexial. Blood pressure is 170/
80 mmHg, with pulse 110/minute in atrial fibrillation. An early dias-
tolic murmur is heard at the left sternal edge and jugular venous
pressure elevated 6 cm. There are bilateral crackles at both lung bases.
Apart from the joint signs of chronic rheumatoid arthritis, the physical
examination is normal.
Investigations show:
Haemoglobin 6.6 g/dl
MCHC 33 g/dl
MCV 110 fl
White cell count 7.4 × 10⁹/l (normal differential)
Platelet count 400 × 10⁹/l
Serum bilirubin 24 μmol/l

Questions:
(1) Give 4 possible causes for her anaemia.
(2) Give 3 causes of her cardiac failure.

Q13 A 59-year-old retired man presents with a 24-hour history of unsteadiness. He smokes 40 cigarettes a day and is a heavy drinker of alcohol. His wife initially thought that he was intoxicated, but began to worry when the unsteadiness persisted. She mentions that he has been slowing up over the previous few months, and for some weeks has been complaining of malaise and lethargy. On specific enquiry he says that he has been deaf in his right ear since World War II, but is otherwise well and has not experienced any tinnitus or vertigo.

The patient is obtunded, afebrile and normotensive. He is wearing a hearing aid in his right ear. Fundoscopy is normal but there is neck stiffness. There is failure of conjugate deviation of the eyes to the right and nystagmus noted with the slow phase directed to the left. There is diminished co-ordination of the right arm and leg with reflexes brisker on the left. When asked to walk the patient consistently falls to the right.

Questions:
Discuss 6 possible diagnoses.

Q14 A 30-year-old female presents with a 2 year history of increasing breathlessness on exertion associated with chest discomfort, weakness and fatigue. She recently developed chest pain on exertion, and was admitted because of an episode of syncope after climbing a flight of stairs at home. She also mentions that her voice has become hoarse. She is a non-smoker and has no complaint of cough, although she admits to 2 episodes of haemoptysis. There is no other significant history.

Examination shows a well looking patient, tachypnoeic at rest. She is apyrexial with no clubbing or cyanosis. The jugular venous pressure is elevated 6 cm and a prominent 'a' wave noted. There is a left parasternal heave and marked systolic pulsation in the second left intercostal space. Auscultation reveals a normal first heart sound, an ejection systolic click, an accentuated second sound which moves normally with respiration and a low pitched mid-diastolic sound maximal on inspiration.

Chest X-ray shows a cardiac diameter of 17 cm and an enlarged main pulmonary artery with clear lung fields. The electrocardiogram shows a P wave in lead II of 0.35 millivolts, a mean frontal QRS axis of +110°, tall R waves and inverted T waves in leads V1, V2 and V3.

Questions:
(1) What is the clinical diagnosis?
(2) What further investigations would you perform to establish its cause?

A 30-year-old man presents with pain in one knee and both ankles. He also has right-sided pleuritic chest pain and admits to urinary frequency associated with supra-pubic discomfort. Fifteen days previously, whilst on holiday alone in Sicily, he had an acute feverish illness characterized by diarrhoea and pain in the right iliac fossa. The stool did not contain blood or mucus and these symptoms settled within 4 days. He denies extra-marital sexual intercourse.

Q15

Examination shows an ill man with a temperature of 37.8°C. He has mild bilateral conjunctivitis, a right-sided pleural rub and normal ankle joints which are painful on passive movement. There is a tense effusion of the left knee which is hot and tender. He is also tender in the right iliac fossa but no mass is palpable. Digital examination of the rectum is normal and sigmoidoscopy shows the mucosa to be hyperaemic.

Initial investigations show:
Haemoglobin 11.5 g/dl
ESR 84 mm/first h
Total white cell count 13.6×10^9/l (neutrophil leucocytosis)
Plasma sodium 141 mmol/l, potassium 3.2 mmol/l, bicarbonate 31 mmol/l, urea 8.6 mmol/l, creatinine 100 μmol/l
Chest radiograph is normal

Questions:
(1) What is the most likely diagnosis?
(2) Name 3 organisms that are known to cause this syndrome.

Q16 A 64-year-old man is admitted to hospital with a 3 month history of central abdominal pain and episodic diarrhoea, the stool occasionally containing blood but no mucus. He admits to episodes of nocturnal sweating for the previous 2 months. He has lost 6 kg in weight over this time and has been anorexic. In World War II he was a prisoner in Malaya and admits to a high daily intake of alcohol since that time. One year prior to admission he developed acute asthma and he is currently taking inhaled steroids and a bronchodilator.

Examination shows an ill looking, confused man. He has firm, non-tender hepatomegaly, a diffusely tender abdomen and a pyrexia varying between 38 and 39°C. Blood pressure is 210/110 mmHg and fundi are normal.

Investigations show:

Haemoglobin 14 g/dl

White cell count $20 \times 10^9/l$, neutrophil leucocytosis with 4% eosinophils

Plasma electrolytes, urea and creatinine normal

Blood cultures × 4 negative

MSU, microscopy and culture normal

Lumbar puncture: pressure normal, CSF examination normal

Chest radiograph, intravenous urogram, barium meal, barium follow-through and barium enema all normal

Questions:
(1) What is the most likely diagnosis?
(2) What is the most useful investigation to confirm this diagnosis?
(3) Give 3 other possible diagnoses.
(4) Give 3 useful investigations to help in the differential diagnosis.

Q17 A 58-year-old woman is admitted having had a generalized convulsion. She was seen 2 months previously by her general practitioner who was called because of left-sided weakness. He found that the weakness had resolved but that her blood pressure was 170/115 mmHg. She mentioned exertional chest pain and admitted smoking 60 cigarettes a day. He advised her to stop smoking and prescribed sub-lingual trinitrin. Two days prior to the convulsion she was awakened, during a dream, by similar chest pain which lasted 35 minutes and did not respond to glyceryl trinitrate. After this she felt non-specifically unwell and while watching television complained of palpitation and had the fit.

She is drowsy but has no focal neurological signs. Axillary temperature is 38.5°C with a pulse of 130/minute irregularly irregular. The jugular venous pulse is elevated 3 cm with only the V wave observed. Blood pressure is 100/60 mmHg in the supine position, and a pericardial friction rub is heard over the praecordium. Crackles are heard bilaterally over the lung bases.

Questions:
(1) What 4 diagnoses would you consider?

A 45-year-old farmer presents with a 6 month history of polyuria, polydipsia, breathlessness on exertion, sweating and generalized headache. His weight has increased by 10 kg over the preceding 2 years. He has recently noted tingling and stiffness of his hands, particularly in the morning and on direct questioning he admits to a loss of libido and impotence for several years.

Q18

Examination shows a large burly man who has signs of mild congestive cardiac failure. His blood pressure is 190/115 mmHg supine, and fundi show arteriovenous crossing changes. Visual fields are full to confrontation. There is diminution of sensation to pin-prick over the lateral three and a half fingers of both hands.

Questions:
(1) What is the diagnosis?
(2) How would you confirm it?
(3) Give 2 possible causes for the polyuria and polydipsia.
(4) What additional investigations would you perform in order to plan management?
(5) What forms of treatment are available for the primary diagnosis?

Q19 A 54-year-old woman presents 2 months after returning to the UK from Singapore where she had lived for the previous 15 years. For 6 months prior to leaving she had had her bowels open 4 or 5 times a day, producing light coloured stools with no blood or mucus. She had lost over 3 kg during this time, and more recently noted generalized aching, depression and ankle swelling. She mentions on direct questioning that she has difficulty in climbing the stairs.

She is clinically anaemic and has peripheral oedema. Abdominal examination is normal. Proximal muscle weakness is noted.

Investigations show:

Hb 10.5 g/dl
Red cells show a dimorphic picture and target cells
WBC 9.5 × 10⁹/l
MCV 78 fl
MCHC 29 g/dl
Plasma electrolytes, urea and creatinine are normal
Albumin 29 g/l, calcium 2.1 mmol/l, phosphate 0.9 mmol/l, alkaline phosphatase 265 U/l
SGPT 18 U/l
Faecal fat excretion is greater than 25 mmol/day

Questions:
(1) What is the most likely diagnosis?
(2) What would be your next investigation?
(3) Outline your further management of this patient.

Q20 A 4-year-old child is brought into Casualty by his grandmother with whom he has been spending the day whilst his parents are away. He was well and active when she first saw him but a few hours later she noted that he was breathless. He then became progressively lethargic and for the 2 hours prior to being seen by the casualty officer had been vomiting.

On examination he is unconscious with a respiratory rate of 35/minute and is febrile (39.5 °C). The pulse is 120/minute and regular, blood pressure 90/50 mmHg. Cardio-vascular, respiratory and abdominal examination are normal and there are no focal neurological signs.

Investigations show:
Hb 13.5 g/dl
White blood count $8.5 \times 10^9/1$ (normal differential)
Plasma sodium 129 mmol/l, potassium 2.9 mmol/l, urea 7 mmol/l,
creatinine 120 μmol/l, bicarbonate 8 mmol/l, glucose 12 mmol/l
Arterial hydrogen ion 75 nmol; Po_2 12.5 kPa, Pco_2 3.1 kPa
Testing of urine showed 1% glycosuria and ketones + +
Urinary pH was 5.0

Questions:
(1) What is the most likely diagnosis?
(2) Give 3 useful investigations.
(3) Suggest 4 therapeutic measures.

Q21

A previously well 54-year-old man developed double vision and failure of abduction of the right eye was noted. A week later he complained of difficulty in swallowing and this progressed so that after a further 2 weeks there was nasal regurgitation of liquid which was particularly distressing because of increased thirst.

Examination shows a well man who is alert and orientated. Visual acuity, optic fundi and pupils are normal with visual fields full to confrontation. The right eye fails to move laterally beyond the midline, and although the movements of the left eye are normal, there is failure of gaze to the right. Facial sensation is intact, but flattening of the right naso-labial fold and the creases of the right forehead is noted. His speech is nasal with no dysarthria. The soft palate deviates to the left and the gag reflex is depressed bilaterally. Shoulder and tongue movements are normal. Power, tone, co-ordination, sensation and reflexes in the limbs are normal and plantar responses are flexor.

Questions:
(1) What is the anatomical distribution of the lesion(s)?
(2) Give 2 possible diagnoses.

Q22 A 62-year-old publican who admits to a daily intake of 10 pints of beer was admitted as an emergency with a leaking aortic aneurysm. Liver function tests on admission were normal. The aneurysm was successfully treated with Dacron grafting and laparotomy was normal. Forty-eight hours later further exploration was required because of continuing haemorrhage. Additional sutures around the graft controlled the bleeding.

Two days after the second operation he was noted to be jaundiced and had a pyrexia of 38.5°C. His pyrexia was thought to be caused by a chest infection and he was treated with physiotherapy and intravenous amoxycillin.

Liver function tests showed:
Serum bilirubin 87 μmol/l
Plasma alkaline phosphatase 320 U/l
SGPT 47 U/l.

Two weeks later he was fit for discharge from hospital and these tests had returned to normal.

He was seen in the surgical clinic 2 months after discharge and was well. Liver function tests showed:
Serum bilirubin 10 μmol/l
Alkaline phosphatase 100 U/l
SGPT 140 U/l.

Two weeks later the patient is seen in the medical clinic. He is well but non-tender enlargement of the liver is noted. Liver function tests now show:
Serum bilirubin 12 μmol/l
Alkaline phosphatase 96 U/l SGPT 200 U/l.

Questions:
(1) What investigations would you perform?
(2) What is the likely diagnosis?

A 25-year-old homosexual man presents with resolving painless jaundice. The illness had started 1 month previously with anorexia and malaise which had improved when jaundice appeared. He had noted pale stools and dark urine. In the previous 6 months he had not left the UK, nor been admitted to hospital and denied taking any drugs.

Q23

Following birth he had had prolonged 'physiological' jaundice which cleared spontaneously at the age of 4 months. There had been a further episode of jaundice at the age of 11 years when firm splenomegaly was noted.

Examination on admission shows a well looking man with no cutaneous stigmata of chronic liver disease. He has slight icterus and a firm spleen palpable 8 cm below the costal margin. The liver is thought not to be clinically enlarged and there is no ascites.

Initial investigations show:

Urine: bile + + + urobilinogen +

Haemoglobin 14.6 g/dl

WBC $8.0 \times 10^9/l$

Plasma urea and electrolytes normal

Prothrombin time 18 seconds, control 14 seconds

Plasma albumin 26 g/l

SGPT 120 U/l

Alkaline phosphatase 200 U/l

Bilirubin 60 μmol/l

Hepatitis B surface antigen positive

Hepatitis Be antigen positive

Hepatitis B antibody negative

^{99}Tc sulphur colloid liver scan shows reduced patchy uptake in a normal sized liver and increased uptake in the bone marrow and spleen.

Questions:
(1) What is the most likely cause of his present illness?
(2) Give 2 diagnostic investigations.

Q24 A 62-year-old man presents with a 2 week history of malaise, anorexia and constant generalized abdominal pain. During this time he has lost 5 kg in weight. For the previous 4 days he had had diarrhoea and vomiting and had been febrile.

During World War II he had served in the Far East where he had had an episode of dysentery. Two years previously, polymyalgia rheumatica had been diagnosed and he had been treated with steroids, the current dose being prednisolone 7.5 mg daily.

He is ill and pyrexial (39°C). The only other abnormal physical finding is tenderness to percussion posteriorly over the right lower chest.

Investigations show:

Haemoglobin 11.2 g/dl

Mean corpuscular volume 80 fl

Mean corpuscular haemoglobin concentration 35 g/dl

White cell count 16×10^9/l (neutrophil leucocytosis)

ESR 110 mm/h

Plasma sodium 128 mmol/l, potassium 3.1 mmol/l, bicarbonate 30 mmol/l, urea 10 mmol/l, creatinine 130 μmol/l

Bilirubin 17 μmol/l

Alkaline phosphatase 200 U/l

SGPT 65 U/l

Total protein 50 g/l

Albumin 20 g/l

Chest radiograph shows a calcified focus in the right mid-zone and a small right pleural effusion

Abdominal radiograph is normal

MSU: no cells, no growth

Stool cultures are negative

Blood cultures grew Gram-positive cocci later identified as *Streptococcus milleri*

Questions:
(1) What is the likely diagnosis?
(2) What further three investigations would you request?
(3) What would be your further management?

A 23-year-old man is brought in by a workmate having collapsed at work. For 48 hours he has been unwell with malaise, myalgia, headache and progressive drowsiness. The patient is unable to give any further history, but his friend mentions that the family suffers from anaemia.

Q25

Examination shows an ill, drowsy, well nourished young man with a pyrexia of 39.8° C. His pulse is 160/minute and blood pressure 75/30 mmHg. Respiratory rate is 28/minute, but there are no focal signs in the chest. There is no abdominal tenderness and he has a well-healed left paramedian scar. There is purpura on the legs and trunk. Examination of fundi is normal and there is no neck-stiffness or focal neurological signs.

An intravenous infusion is set up but his blood pressure fails to respond to fluid and colloid replacement. The infusion site continues to bleed.

Initial investigation show:

Haemoglobin 10.4 g/dl

Total white blood cell count 3.4×10^9/l (95% lymphocytes)

Platelets 270×10^9/l

Plasma sodium 119 mmol/l, potassium 3.1 mmol/l, bicarbonate 17 mmol/l, glucose 1.5 mmol/l, urea 6.5 mmol/l, creatinine 150 μmol/l

A lumbar puncture is performed and this shows clear cerebro-spinal fluid. Microscopy shows 12 red cells and no white cells. Biochemistry shows glucose of 3.5 mmol/l and protein of 0.2 g/l. No organisms are seen.

Questions:

(1) What is the diagnosis?

(2) Suggest possible causes.

(3) What is the cause of:

    (a) The bleeding tendency.

    (b) The low blood glucose.

    (c) The granulocytopenia.

    (d) The hyponatraemia.

Q26 A 55-year-old widower who lives alone in poor social circumstances presents with a 4 month history of weakness, weight loss and diffuse musculo–skeletal pain. He is a heavy smoker and on the day of presentation had sharp left-sided chest pain following a bout of severe coughing.

Examination shows a thin dishevelled man with a distended abdomen and mild bilateral proptosis. No lymph nodes are palpable and the thyroid gland is normal. There is increased antero-posterior diameter of the chest and tenderness of the left 5th rib anteriorly. Respiratory movements are limited by pain and there are coarse crackles and wheezes over the thorax. There is no evidence of ascites, the liver is palpable but soft and smooth. The bowel sounds are increased. Apart from weakness of the shoulder and pelvic girdle muscles, neurological examination is normal. Walking is difficult because of generalized pain.

Initial investigations show:

Haemoglobin 10.2 g/dl

White blood count 9.0×10^9/l

MCV 100 fl

MCHC 35 g/dl

ESR 40 mm/h

Plasma electrolytes, urea and creatinine normal

Serum calcium 2.2 mmol/l, albumin 32 g/l, phosphate 0.7 mmol/l, alkaline phosphatase 650 U/l

SGPT 30 U/l

CPK 200 U/l

Chest radiograph shows a fracture of the left 5th rib anteriorly and erosion of the distal ends of the clavicles. Low flat diaphragms are also noted.

Question:

Give 5 useful investigations.

Answers:

A1

(1) The combination of high fever, agitation, diarrhoea, an irregular tachycardia and hypercalcaemia suggests a diagnosis of thyroid storm. Support for this diagnosis comes from the preceding history of weight loss and diarrhoea and the family history of organ-specific autoimmune disease. Addison's disease may present with diarrhoea and abdominal pain but the electrolytes are against this diagnosis. The serum albumin should be low for malabsorption to be considered as a likely diagnosis.

(2) (a) Thyroid hormone level. It should be emphasized that thyroid crisis is a clinical diagnosis and the serum thyroxine is no higher than in 'ordinary' thyrotoxicosis. Treatment may have to be started before this result is obtained.

(b) A thyroid uptake scan to detect increased early uptake.

(3) Thyroid storm (or crisis) usually occurs as a result of stress such as infection, in a patient whose thyrotoxicosis is poorly controlled. Patients may, however, present in thyroid crisis.

The management of this condition is as follows:

(a) Supportive treatment which consists of cooling, sedation, intravenous fluids and nasogastric aspiration if the patient is vomiting.

(b) Specific treatment to inhibit thyroidal production of T4 and T3, peripheral production of T3, and the peripheral actions of thyroid hormones. Propylthiouracil (250 mg six-hourly orally or via a nasogastric tube) has the theoretical advantage over carbimazole in that as well as inhibiting synthesis of T4 and T3 it also inhibits peripheral conversion of T4 to T3. Lugol's Iodine (5% iodine, 10% potassium iodide) 30 drops per day in divided doses, reduces thyroidal hormone synthesis. Alternatively, potassium iodide 1 to 2 g per day may be given intravenously. Propranolol 1 to 5 mg intravenously six-hourly reduces the peripheral manifestations of the thyroid hormones.

A2

Answers:

(1) This girl has features which enable the diagnosis of Toxic Shock Syndrome to be made. Detailed descriptions of the criteria for this diagnosis are given in the 2 references. The criteria include:

(a) Pyrexia

(b) Rash with desquamation 1–2 weeks after the onset of the illness

(c) Evidence of shock: systolic blood pressure less than 90 mmHg in adults, or symptoms of postural hypotension.

(d) Clinical or laboratory evidence of involvement of 3 or more organ systems. Most patients have gastro-intestinal symptoms with vomiting and diarrhoea. Biochemical tests of liver function may be abnormal and there may be evidence of renal failure. Other common symptoms are myalgia and disorientation.

(e) Blood and CSF cultures should be negative.

(2) Management is initially directed towards reversing the shock with intravenous fluid replacement. The pathogenesis in the syndrome has not been fully established, but a toxin produced by *Staphylococcus aureus* and absorbed from or via the vagina has been implicated. Treatment with beta-lactamase-resistant antibiotics has been advocated.

The incidence of recurrence of the syndrome is thought to be reduced by the use of appropriate antibiotics in the treatment of the acute illness. The patient should discontinue the use of tampons for several menstrual cycles afterwards, and be advised against their extended use. She should be advised to report promptly any untoward symptoms occurring at the time of menstruation.

References

Davis, J. P., Chesney, P. J., Wand, P. J., and LaVenture, M. (1980). Toxic Shock Syndrome: Epidemiologic Features, Recurrence, Risk factors, and Prevention. *New Engl. J. Med.*, 303, 1429–1435

Shands, K. N., Schmid, G. P., Dan, B. B. et al. (1980). Toxic Shock Syndrome in Menstruating Women: Association with Tampon Use and Staphylococcus aureus and Clinical Features in 52 cases. *New Engl. J. Med.*, 303, 1436–1442

Answers:
(1) Her symptoms are due to postural hypotension as there is a fall of **A3** systolic blood pressure of more than 30 mmHg from supine to standing position. Two possible mechanisms are:
  (a) Excessive diuretic therapy leading to a reduction in intravascular volume. The relatively normal plasma creatinine, elevated urea and the electrolytes would strongly support this diagnosis.
  (b) Diabetic autonomic neuropathy. She has been an insulin-requiring diabetic for 10 years and has background retinopathy and absent ankle reflexes.
(2) (a) Discontinue diuretic therapy and assess symptomatic response. It would be possible to give an intravenous infusion of physiological saline, but in the presence of myocardial insufficiency this may precipitate heart failure.
  (b) Investigate the possibility of autonomic neuropathy by demonstrating abnormal cardiovascular responses to stress.

  A standard test is the performance of Valsalva's manoeuvre (maintenance of a column of mercury to 40 mm for 15 seconds) with simultaneous recording of the electrocardiogram. The ratio of the longest R–R interval after the manoeuvre to the shortest during the manoeuvre will be less than 1.1:1 in patients with autonomic neuropathy.

  Further tests include response to sustained hand grip and measurement of beat-to-beat variation on the electrocardiogram. The comparison of resting supine heart rate to the heart rate recorded 15 beats after assuming the standing position is a similar test.
(3) (a) Reduction in diuretic therapy should produce symptomatic relief
  (b) (i) Antigravity stockings
    (ii) 9 alpha-fludrocortisone
    (iii) Sympathomimetic therapy (such as ephedrine)
    (iv) Indomethacin has been used with some success (anti-prostaglandin activity)
    (v) Vaso-constriction using ergot preparations (dihydroergotamine) is useful, but should be avoided in this patient because of vascular disease.

The 5-year survival of diabetics with automonic neuropathy is reduced by 50 per cent. The identification of diabetic patients with autonomic neuropathy is also useful in predicting those who will have an abnormal cardiovascular response to general anaesthesia.

A4 Answers:

(1) Guillain–Barré syndrome. This usually presents as ascending paralysis, and in half the cases there is a history of preceding infection which has cleared by the time the manifestations of neuropathy appear. The weakness is usually symmetrical, beginning in the legs and associated with areflexia. Sensory loss is variable. There is often sphincter involvement and muscle pain is present in approximately 30% of patients, but less severe than in poliomyelitis. There may also be features of autonomic dysfunction. Cerebro-spinal fluid protein is elevated and usually there is no increase in cells.

The CSF results obtained suggest a traumatic tap, the proportion of red cells to white cells being the same as in the peripheral blood (approximately 500:1). There is, therefore, no increase in inflammatory cells. The protein is markedly elevated and cannot be accounted for by the presence of increased red cells (the presence of 700 red cells/mm³ causes an elevation of CSF protein of approximately 1 mg). This raised CSF protein in the absence of a cellular response is characteristic of Guillain–Barré syndrome.

(2) and (3)

(a) Poliomyelitis is suggested by the history except for the fact that there is no evidence of clinical meningitis. The weakness of poliomyelitis is usually asymmetrical and involves the larger proximal muscle groups. It is extremely unusual to have impaired sensation in poliomyelitis, and the muscle pain is usually greater than that described in this case. There would be an increase in the inflammatory cells in the CSF suggesting a lymphocytic meningitis.

(b) A cauda equina lesion is suggested by the flaccid paralysis and sphincter involvement in association with back pain. The narrowing of the L4 disc space as shown on the radiograph possibly suggests disc prolapse as a cause of the neurological deficit, but the radiological appearances, particularly in the elderly, are non-specific. Spinal cord block would cause greatly elevated CSF protein in the absence of cellular response

(Froin's syndrome). It would be important to document that CSF pressure varies with respiration. Against this diagnosis is the minimal loss of sensation and no evidence of sensory level. It would also be difficult to fit distal weakness in the arms with a cauda equina lesion. Two other conditions to consider are:

(a) Myasthenia gravis, which may be excluded by a tensilon test
(b) Acute polymyositis (which may be excluded by a normal plasma creatine kinase estimation).

Answers:

A5

(1) The history strongly suggests a diagnosis of fasting hypoglycaemia. Investigations should be directed firstly towards proving spontaneous hypoglycaemia; secondly establishing the presence of organic hyperinsulinism and thirdly to determining its cause. The following would be appropriate investigations:

(a) A prolonged fast of up to 72 hours with blood taken for glucose and insulin estimation if there are any symptoms suggestive of hypoglycaemia. Fasting blood may be taken for blood glucose and plasma insulin estimations, and a high insulin to glucose ratio would be expected in organic hyperinsulinism. However, elevated serum insulin in the presence of spontaneous hypoglycaemia is better.

(b) C-peptide suppression test. This is measurement of C-peptide during hypoglycaemia induced by intravenous purified insulin. Failure to completely suppress C-peptide production suggests endogenous inappropriate production of insulin, and this is most likely to be due to an insulinoma. Investigations should then proceed to localize the tumour by coeliac axis angiography, or percutaneous transhepatic catheterization of the splenic and portal veins with blood sampling for insulin. Abdominal CT scanning is unlikely to be useful because of the small size of the tumour. Measurement of C-peptide during spontaneous hypoglycaemia is also useful as suppression suggests an exogenous source of insulin.

(2) The symptoms suggest recurrent hypoglycaemia associated with

fasting or exercise. Weight-gain is an important consequence of recurrent hypoglycaemia. Her profession, a close relative with insulin-dependent diabetes mellitus, and past and recent psychiatric trouble, strongly suggest factitious hypoglycaemia as a cause of her symptoms. However, many patients with insulinoma have an abnormal mental state. A feature of patients who have factitious hypoglycaemia is that they tend to produce symptoms at a time likely to cause maximum attention.

On balance it is likely that she has an insulinoma, but factitious hypoglycaemia is a strong possibility.

A6

Answers:
(1) There is pancytopenia with no abnormal cells but a macrocytosis. The raised mean corpuscular volume could be explained by phenytoin therapy, reticulocytosis or a megaloblastic process due to vitamin B_{12} deficiency.

The possible causes for the haematological abnormalities are:
(a) Paroxysmal nocturnal haemoglobinuria (PNH) suggested by previous episodes of back pain and dark urine. PNH often terminates in an aplastic process and reticulocytosis would be a feature of haemolysis (although not present with bone marrow aplasia).
(b) 'Idiopathic' aplastic anaemia.
(c) Aplastic anaemia following viral hepatitis. This is well documented and many causes of 'idiopathic' aplastic anaemia may be post-viral.
(d) Aleukaemic leukaemia. Patients with Down's Syndrome have a 10–20 fold increase in acute leukaemia. The cell types follow the usual distribution, but the age peak is earlier and the presentation is usually during the first decade of life.
(e) Vitamin B_{12} deficiency.

(2) Examination of a bone marrow aspirate would give most information at this stage. This may show a megaloblastic process (vitamin B_{12} deficiency), the presence of leukaemic blast cells or aplasia.

Answers:

This is an elderly man with an elevated erythrocyte sedimentation rate, nephrotic syndrome, hepatomegaly and abnormal immunoglobulin production.

Disorders associated with monoclonal immunoglobulin production are:

(a) multiple myeloma

(b) macroglobulinaemia

(c) amyloidosis

(d) benign monoclonal gammopathy (there should be no immuno-suppression, no overproduction of light chains, total amount of protein less than 10 g/l, no increase in amount of protein with time)

(e) B-cell neoplasms (chronic lymphatic leukaemia and non-Hodgkin's lymphoma)

(f) non-lymphoid neoplasms (carcinoma of colon and breast)

(g) some conditions associated with hypergammaglobulinaemia

(1) Three possible diagnoses are:

(a) Amyloid. Infiltration with amyloid material would explain nephrotic syndrome, hepatomegaly and low voltage electrocardiogram. Amyloid is a condition in which there is overproduction of immunoglobulin and this may result in an M-band and even immune suppression. The diagnosis may be confirmed by histological examination of biopsy specimens from involved organs (liver and kidney in this case) or from rectum or gingiva.

(b) Myeloma. In addition to overproduction of abnormal immunoglobulins it is necessary to demonstrate malignant plasma cells (bone marrow aspiration or trephine biopsy) and typical lytic lesions of bone. This is best done by a skeletal survey rather than a bone scan.

(c) Malignancy, particularly of the large bowel. This may be associated with an M-band and immune paresis. The nephrotic syndrome may be due to membranous glomerulonephritis associated with malignancy, and the hepatomegaly to secondary deposits within the liver.

(2) Useful investigations would be:

(a) biopsy of liver, kidney, rectum or gum

(b) bone marrow aspiration or trephine biopsy

(c) skeletal survey

(d) ⁹⁹Tc sulphur colloid liver scan
(e) barium enema

A8 **Answers:**
(1) Liver failure. Although the presentation is that of central nervous system disturbance, the normal lumbar puncture makes a metabolic cause likely. Liver failure is suggested by the reversal of sleep pattern, the low plasma sodium and the low plasma urea. An overdose of the tricyclic antidepressant is a possibility but the absence of tachycardia and dilated pupils makes this less likely.
(2) (a) alcoholic liver disease.
   (b) haemochromatosis – suggested by 'suntan', arthritis and diabetes.
   (c) acute viral hepatitis.
   (d) paracetamol overdose.
(3) (a) Biochemical tests of liver function (bilirubin, enzymes, albumin and clotting screen) will be useful in confirming the clinical diagnosis of hepatic coma. Of these the SGPT should distinguish acute fulminant hepatitis (very high) from chronic liver disease.
   (b) serum ferritin. This is raised in iron overload.
   (c) Serum iron will be high in haemochromatosis with saturation of iron binding protein (70–90%), but may also be elevated in alcoholic liver disease, particularly if there is excessive consumption of red wine. Serum iron would be low in the presence of acute infection or neoplasia (hepatoma being especially relevant in this case).
   (d) a percutaneous liver biopsy would help in the diagnosis of acute hepatitis and may show iron overload. The secondary iron overload that occurs in patients with alcohol induced liver disease is usually less than that seen in haemochromatosis, but the difference is often not sufficient to be diagnostic.
   (e) quantitation of urinary iron excretion following administration of desferrioxamine. This is a good measure of the degree of iron overload and helps to separate primary from secondary.

Answers:

(1) There is a hypokalaemic alkalosis with an elevated urea and creatinine. This may be caused by:
- (a) Diarrhoea. Either secondary to magnesium-containing antacids, or a side-effect of antihypertensive treatment (propranolol or methyldopa). A further possible cause is purgative abuse (he is known to manipulate his own medication).
- (b) Diuretic therapy.
- (c) Carbenoxolone may cause salt and water retention with hypokalaemia. This may have been self-administered for his peptic ulceration. Excessive consumption of liquorice (from the sweet shop) may produce the same effect.
- (d) Ectopic production of ACTH from a bronchial carcinoma. He is a middle-aged man who is a heavy cigarette smoker and has a history of dry cough and weight loss. Cushingoid features are often not present in this syndrome as death occurs before they develop.
- (e) Conn's syndrome.

The elevated urea and creatinine may be caused by dehydration associated with polyuria or diarrhoea, but persistant hypokalaemia itself may cause renal impairment. The alkalosis is a feature of hypokalaemia but may be increased by antacid therapy.

(2) Possible causes for polyuria include:
- (a) Hypokalaemia causing renal tubular damage.
- (b) Hypercalcaemia from carcinoma of the bronchus (with lytic bony deposits; if the abnormal biochemistry were caused by ACTH production, this would suggest an oat cell tumour - it is a squamous cell tumour that produces PTH) or due to the milk-alkali syndrome.
- (c) Diuretic therapy.

Answers:

(1) Pleural biopsy (Abram's needle). Biopsy of the pleura at the time of aspiration of fluid is useful in the diagnosis of malignant or tuberculous pleural effusion. Histological confirmation of the diagnosis is obtained in 40–60% of cases of malignant disease and up

to 80% of cases of tuberculosis. Sampling from different areas may be required.

(2) This patient's occupational history suggests prolonged exposure to asbestos, and the pleural thickening seen on the chest radiograph is consistent with this. His history of several years increasing breathlessness is unlikely to be due to the pleural effusion but may be due to interstitial lung disease. There are, however, no radiographic or clinical signs to support this.

With the decline of primary tuberculous infection in the UK pleural effusion has become less common, and now occurs most frequently in older patients who may not have pulmonary lesions. In this patient the cytological findings (mesothelial cells with relatively few lymphocytes) in the pleural fluid are against this diagnosis.

Likely diagnoses, therefore are:

(a) bronchial carcinoma – increased six-fold following exposure to asbestos with a 20–30 year latent period. In a cigarette smoker the risk rises to 100 times that of the general population.

(b) malignant mesothelioma – occurs in 3% of asbestos workers who have not been protected against exposure and on average occurs 40 years after exposure.

A11 Answers:

(1) This is a middle-aged woman with a goitre who is biochemically hypothyroid and has hypercalcaemia. Possible diagnoses are:

(a) Hashimoto's thyroiditis. Hypercalcaemia may rarely be a feature of hypothyroidism. Such patients have reduced tolerance of an oral calcium load, possibly due to retarded incorporation of calcium into bone.

(b) Follicular carcinoma of the thyroid. This characteristically occurs in middle-aged women and may metastasize to bone, causing lytic lesions and the possibility of hypercalcaemia. Papillary carcinoma tends to occur in a younger age group and not to metastasize to bone.

(c) Medullary carcinoma of the thyroid. This may be associated with hyperparathyroidism as part of the multiple endocrine adenoma syndrome (type II). Medullary carcinoma accounts for about 10% of cases of thyroid carcinoma and is probably under-diagnosed.

(2) (a) Thyroid scan. Diffuse irregular patchy distribution of tracer suggests thyroiditis (rarely anaplastic carcinoma). An area of failure of uptake ('cold nodule') suggests malignancy.

(b) Thyroid auto-antibodies. These are present in high titres in over 90% of patients with Hashimoto's thyroiditis. Lower titres are found in other thyroid diseases.

(c) Serum calcitonin level. This is a very good marker for medullary carcinoma. Measure either the basal level or that following stimulation with ethanol orally or pentagastrin intravenously.

(3) (a) Thyroxine replacement.

(b) Follicular carcinoma will require surgery (total or near-total thyroidectomy) for diagnosis and treatment. Radio-active iodine (^{131}I) is injected intravenously about 2 weeks after surgery followed by total body scintiscan to look for uptake in metastases. This may occur despite non-uptake by the primary tumour. Metastases are treated with an ablative dose of ^{131}I. Following this treatment is with L-thyroxine in a dose sufficient to completely suppress TSH, as the tumour may be TSH-dependent. Oral thyroxine replacement is changed to triiodothyronine (a much shorter half life) every 3 months during the first year and this is withdrawn in order to repeat the scan. A further dose of radio-active iodine may be required.

(c) Total thyroidectomy is indicated for treatment of proven medullary carcinoma of the thyroid. The patient and relatives should be screened for associated tumours - pheochromocytoma and hyperplasia of the parathyroids.

Answers:

(1) (a) Haemolytic anaemia. This is suggested by the normal MCHC, raised MCV suggesting reticulocytosis and elevated bilirubin. Possible causes of this are:

A12

(i) Auto-immune, either secondary to drug therapy (methyldopa) or idiopathic.

(ii) Glucose-6-phosphate dehydrogenase deficiency (in view of her ethnic background).

      (iii) Associated with lymphoma. The patient has generalized pruritus but this may be a feature of severe anaemia *per se.*

  (b) Megaloblastic anaemia. Pernicious anaemia is associated with rheumatoid arthritis. However, the white cell count and platelet count are normal and there is no splenomegaly.

  (c) Hypothyroidism may cause a macrocytic normoblastic anaemia and also cardiac failure.

  (d) Infective endocarditis must be considered in the presence of anaemia and a murmur suggestive of aortic regurgitation, but this is usually associated with a normochromic normocytic anaemia and a neutrophil leucocytosis.

(2) Possible causes of this patient's cardiac failure are:

  (a) Anaemia.

  (b) Hypertension.

  (c) Ischaemic heart disease. This may be either atheromatous (long-standing hypertension) or may be due to rheumatoid arteritis of the coronary arteries.

  (d) Aortic incompetence, either secondary to hypertension or possibly infective endocarditis.

  (e) Cardiomyopathy, this is suggested by congestive heart failure and atrial fibrillation in the absence of obvious cause. Rheumatoid arthritis is the commonest cause of amyloidosis in the United Kingdom and although secondary cardiac amyloid is rare, this may be a possible cause of the cardiomyopathy. Rheumatoid disease may cause a myocarditis leading to cardiac failure. Chronic alcohol abuse is a cause of macrocytosis and congestive cardiomyopathy.

A13

Answers:

There is a history of malaise and lethargy and a short history of gait disturbance. The physical signs are those of a right cerebellar hemisphere lesion. The following diagnoses should be considered:

(1) Cerebellar abscess. The commonest cause of this is direct extension from infection of the middle ear, mastoid or nasal air sinuses. There is often a latent interval of weeks or months following an exacerbation of otitis before the signs of abscess appear. There

may be sub-occipital headache which radiates down the neck associated with cervical rigidity. Signs of cerebellar dysfunction vary in severity and may be slight.

It is important to question this patient about the cause of his deafness and about any discharge from the ear, and it is imperative to remove the hearing aid to allow full auroscopic examination.

This patient had a chronically discharging ear, and a skull radiograph showed obliteration of the mastoid air space and sclerosis of the petrous bone. A cranial CT scan showed an abscess of the right cerebellar hemisphere.

(2) Cerebellar hemisphere secondary from carcinoma of the bronchus.

(3) Cerebellar haemorrhage. Such patients have a sudden onset of symptoms, often with vomiting, and a proportion of cases are unconscious on admission. Only a minority of patients have localizing signs, and repeated vomiting and vertigo in an ataxic patient should suggest this diagnosis. If a cerebellar haemorrhage is confirmed, surgical evacuation should be considered.

The signs and symptoms in this case are unlikely to be due to the lateral medullary syndrome as there are no sensory signs, and long tract involvement is usually more prominent.

(4) Acoustic neuroma. The presentation is usually with symptoms due to disturbance of function of the 8th cranial nerve. Tinnitus is usually followed by progressive deafness and there may also be labyrinthine symptoms. In this patient the duration of deafness would be against this diagnosis.

(5) Alcoholic cerebellar degeneration. This usually affects both hemispheres and also the vermis. It is characterized by ataxia but nystagmus is unusual.

(6) Sub-acute cerebellar degeneration secondary to a neoplasm (usually a non-metastatic complication of carcinoma of the bronchus). This usually presents with rapidly progressive bilateral cerebellar signs.

(7) Hypothyroidism. This may present with cerebellar ataxia.

In general the differential diagnosis of cerebellar syndromes should also include hereditary degeneration (often spino-cerebellar) and phenytoin toxicity.

47

A14

Answers:

(1) Pulmonary hypertension. The recurrent laryngeal nerve may be compressed by the dilated pulmonary artery causing the hoarse voice. The mid-diastolic sound is likely to be a right ventricular third sound but may be caused by mitral stenosis.

(2) The following are the main causes of pulmonary hypertension:

    (a) primary

    (b) congenital heart disease, particularly atrial septal defect

    (c) recurrent pulmonary emboli (thrombus, fat or schistosoma)

    (d) systemic collagen diseases such as scleroderma, systemic lupus erythematosus

    (e) sarcoidosis

    (f) left atrial and pulmonary venous hypertension often secondary to heart valve disease, particularly mitral stenosis

    (g) chronic lung disease (e.g. lung fibrosis or occupational lung disease)

    (h) alveolar hypoventilation

The history, physical examination and chest radiograph will exclude most of the above. The following investigations may be needed for a diagnosis of mitral stenosis, atrial septal defect or recurrent pulmonary emboli:

    (a) ventilation and perfusion lung scan

    (b) echocardiography

    (c) pulmonary angiography – to exclude pulmonary emboli, and to document and quantitate the pulmonary hypertension and measure pulmonary wedge pressure

    (d) lung function tests

    (e) a lung biopsy is sometimes required although great care should be taken in the presence of raised pulmonary artery pressure

---

A15

Answers:

(1) Reactive arthritis following an episode of dysentery (Reiter's syndrome). Reiter's original description in 1916 was of a Cavalry officer who developed an acute dysenteric illness characterized by urethritis, arthritis and conjunctivitis. In the UK and USA, most cases follow extra-marital sexual intercourse, whereas in Europe dysentery is more frequently the precipitating event. In post-dysen-

teric Reiter's disease, arthritis begins between 1–3 weeks (average 15 days) after the initial symptoms which tend to be mild. Weight-bearing joints, particularly knees and ankles, are involved asymmetrically and may be associated with effusion. An important differential diagnosis is gonococcal arthritis, and if any doubt exists aspiration of joint fluid should be performed. The primary gonococcal infection in non-homosexual men is usually symptomatic. The urethritis of Reiter's syndrome is usually mild and may be detected by noting strands of mucus in the 'two glass' urine test. Ocular and skin lesions are characteristic and other rarer manifestations include pleurisy.

(2) (i) *Shigella flexneri*
(ii) *Salmonella typhimurium*
(iii) *Yersinia enterocolitica* – particularly associated with terminal ileitis as in this case
(iv) *Campylobacter* has recently been reported to cause the syndrome
(v) there are case reports of amoebic dysentery being followed by Reiter's syndrome

Brucella may cause a similar clinical picture but preceding dysenteric illness is absent.

Answers:
(1) Polyarteritis nodosa (PAN). This is an elderly man with a systemic disease, the features of which include pyrexia, weight loss, abdominal symptoms, asthma, hypertension and a leucocytosis with eosinophilia. These strongly suggest a diagnosis of PAN. **A16**

(2) The diagnosis of PAN may be difficult to confirm. In the presence of haematuria a renal biopsy is useful. A non-selective skin or muscle biopsy may show evidence of arteritis but the yield is higher if the muscle chosen is painful. Perhaps the most useful investigation is coeliac axis angiography which may show the characteristic aneurysms up to 1 cm in size. These are seen in the visceral vasculature in up to 80% of cases. Hepatitis B surface antigen is found in about 20% of patients with PAN.

(3) The differential diagnosis includes those causes of pyrexia of unknown origin (PUO) with abdominal symptoms.

(a) lymphoma (particularly Hodgkin's disease with eosinophilia).
(b) intra-abdominal abscess, particularly sub-phrenic and hepatic (pyogenic or amoebic - prisoner in Malaya).
(c) a hepatoma developing in a cirrhotic liver.
(d) tuberculosis. A normal chest radiograph does not exclude this, but a normal lumbar puncture makes tuberculous meningitis unlikely.
(e) Whipple's disease.
(f) Crohn's disease is unlikely in view of the normal barium studies.

(4) (a) computed tomography of the abdomen.
(b) ultrasound of the liver and sub-phrenic areas.
(c) ^{99}Tc sulphur-colloid liver scan.
(d) sputum smears for acid fast bacilli (the tuberculin skin test may be negative in 10–40% of patients with miliary tuberculosis).

A17

Answers:
This is a middle-aged woman with vascular disease (angina and transient cerebral ischaemic attack) associated with hypertension and heavy cigarette smoking. She presents with a generalized convulsion, hypotension, atrial fibrillation (irregular pulse and absent 'a' wave in the jugular venous pulse) and pericarditis. She has a fever but this may be due to the fit. There is also mild heart failure. Diagnoses to consider are:

(1) myocardial infarction sustained during the episode of nocturnal pain. Although rest pain should be considered as infarction it is possible to have angina 'at rest' when asleep, the pain being precipitated by vascular response to dreaming. The infarct may have caused a fall in blood pressure which would be exacerbated by the onset of atrial fibrillation (suggested by the palpitation). Hypotension in the presence of cerebro-vascular disease may lead to an hypoxic convulsion. Fever, pericarditis and heart failure are common complications of myocardial infarction.

(2) collagen disease. Pericarditis and cerebral involvement occur particularly in systemic lupus erythematosus. The pyrexia could be due to the disease and the hypotension due to myocardial infarction possibly associated with coronary arteritis.

(3) bronchial neoplasm. This could cause atrial fibrillation and peri-carditis as a result of local involvement of the pericardium and a generalized convulsion due to cerebral secondary deposits. The fall in blood pressure may be caused by pericardial effusion but the venous pressure was not noted to rise paradoxically with respiration.

(4) uraemia causing a fit and pericardial friction rub. The hypotension may be due to myocardial infarction or due to decreased intra-vascular volume associated with dehydration.

(5) infective endocarditis should be considered as a cause of stroke, myocardial infarction and pyrexia.

(6) viral encephalitis associated with viral pericarditis should also be considered.

Answers:

(1) Acromegaly.

(2) Failure of suppression of growth hormone, measured by radio-immunoassay, during an oral glucose tolerance test.

(3) (a) Glycosuria from diabetes mellitus.

    (b) Hypercalciuria - acromegaly may be associated with hyper-parathyroidism but growth hormone also stimulates the for-mation of 1,25 dihydroxycholecalciferol leading to increased calcium absorption from the gut.

    (c) Possibly diabetes insipidus. It is unusual for a growth-hormone-secreting pituitary tumour to involve the hypo-thalamus and cause diabetes insipidus.

(4) Investigations should be directed towards determining the follow-ing:

    (a) The size and degree of suprasellar extension of the tumour.

       (i) Skull radiograph with views of the pituitary fossa (tom-ography).

      (ii) Cranial CT scan.

     (iii) Formal perimetry of visual fields.

     (iv) If doubt still exists regarding supra-sellar extension, further neuroradiology is indicated (for example, a con-trast study to outline the tumour).

A18

(b) The effect of the tumour on other anterior pituitary hormones.
  (i) Insulin tolerance test with measurement of cortisol response.
  (ii) TRH test to assess TSH and prolactin.
  (iii) LHRH test.
(c) The extent of growth-hormone-induced tissue over-growth.
  (i) Hand volume measurement by plethysmography.
  (ii) Facial stereo photographs.
  (iii) Heel pad thickness.
  These measurements are useful in assessing the response to treatment.
(d) The presence and severity of complications, for example:
  (i) Electrocardiogram – hypertension, cardiomyopathy.
  (ii) Lung function tests.
  (iii) Assessment of carbohydrate tolerance (oral GTT performed for diagnosis).
(5) Opinions vary as to the best treatment for acromegaly and the following are used:
  (a) Transfrontal hypophysectomy (with or without external irradiation). Most would agree that this is the treatment of choice if there is significant suprasellar extension of the tumour.
  (b) Transsphenoidal hypophysectomy.
  (c) Interstitial irradiation with yttrium.
  (d) External irradiation.
  (e) Bromocriptine (rarely used as definitive treatment).

A19 Answers:

(1) Coeliac disease. History, examination and investigation suggest malabsorption. The associated metabolic bone disease may cause the generalized aches and proximal myopathy. Coeliac disease is the most likely diagnosis, particularly when the dimorphic red cells and target cells (hyposplenism) are considered.
(2) *Per oral* (Crosby capsule) jejunal biopsy. Barium followthrough would confirm the diagnosis of malabsorption but not add to the diagnosis.
(3) Clinical, biochemical and histological improvement should occur with a gluten-free diet, although this may not be evident for some

months. If the patient does not respond to strict exclusion of gluten from the diet the following must be considered:

(a) Concurrent pancreatic insufficiency.
(b) Ileal or jejunal ulceration (with protein-losing enteropathy).
(c) Lactase deficiency.
(d) Intestinal lymphoma.

A diagnosis of tropical sprue is unlikely as this condition should improve rather than worsen following return to the United Kingdom. Although prevalent in large areas in the Far East it is said not to occur in Singapore.

Answers:

A20

(1) This is a child with severe metabolic acidosis who presented with hyperpnoea and then vomiting. The most likely cause in a previously well child is salicylate poisoning, particularly when the child is staying away from home where tablets may not be kept out of reach. Salicylate poisoning causes an initial stimulation of the respiratory centre leading to hyperpnoea, but then a profound metabolic acidosis with vomiting and dehydration, confusion, hyperpyrexia and coma ensue. The hyponatraemia, hypokalaemia and hyperglycaemia are compatible with this diagnosis (the latter a result of increased glycogenolysis and diminished synthesis). The following conditions should also be considered:

(a) Diabetes mellitus. This would cause greater ketonuria if the child were unconscious from ketoacidosis.
(b) Lactic acidosis. When this causes coma in children there are usually preceding neurological problems (or else the presentation is in the neonatal period).
(c) Renal tubular acidosis is unlikely because of the history and low urinary pH.
(d) Encephalitis.

(2) (a) The urine should be boiled to remove ketones and then tested with ferric chloride. If salicylate is present the urine turns red-brown. Alternatively, a positive reaction with Phenistix may be obtained.
(b) Quantitative estimation of plasma salicylate.
(c) Lumbar puncture.

(3) (a) Gastric lavage with endotracheal tube.
    (b) Intravenous infusion of fluids containing sodium and potassium. This will help correct dehydration due to vomiting and hyperpnoea, and will also produce a diuresis which will encourage renal excretion of salicylate.
    (c) Sodium bicarbonate should be included in the fluid regimen, the dosage being adjusted to avoid hypernatraemia and alkalosis and to make urine alkaline. This will correct the severe acidosis and also increase renal tubular excretion of salicylate.
    (d) Administration of Vitamin K_1 to correct prothrombin deficiency and prevent haemorrhage.
    (e) If oliguria is present or there is no improvement in the general state, peritoneal or haemodialysis should be considered.

A21

Answers:
(1) The dysphagia and palatal abnormality indicate a lesion of both 10th cranial nerves or their nuclei, the right being more involved than the left. There is facial weakness of lower motor neurone distribution suggesting a lesion of the 7th nerve or its nucleus. The 6th nerve palsy is unlikely to be nuclear as it is associated with failure of conjugate gaze.
The lesions are in the brain stem and are discrete because:
    (a) There is no involvement of the 5th nerve (near the 6th).
    (b) The 12th nerve is spared and this is at the same level as the 10th nerve nucleus and lies between it and the pyramidal tract.
(2) The approach to defining the pathological process causing these lesions is best done systematically:
    (a) Vascular – the anatomical distribution is against this, as is the time course.
    (b) Demyelination – unlikely as there is no evidence of white matter involvement.
    (c) Infection – brain stem viral encephalitis is rare but may produce this clinical picture. The slow progression is rather against this diagnosis.
    (d) Tumour – a single expanding lesion associated with oedema (such as a glioma) would not produce this patchy involvement.

Gliomas of the brain stem usually involve the pyramidal tract. Lymphoma or multiple secondary deposits are possibilities.

(e) 'Inflammatory processes' – collagen vascular disease or sarcoidosis. The latter involves the brain stem patchily with a predilection for the 7th nerve and hypothalamus. Sarcoidosis in this situation may cause diabetes insipidus (note that this patient complained of increased thirst).

Degenerative, toxic, metabolic and endocrine disorders are not relevant to the discussion of this case.

Possible diagnoses therefore, are:

(a) Lymphoma or secondary deposits infiltrating the brain stem.
(b) Sarcoidosis.
(c) Brain stem encephalitis.

Answers:

This man who has had 2 major operations, presumably requiring blood transfusions, developed a transient mild obstructive jaundice shortly after the second operation. By the time of discharge liver function tests were normal. A few months later the liver function tests showed a hepatitic picture. Possible causes are:

A22

(1) Alcohol. Liver function tests on admission were normal and it is likely that his alcohol ingestion post-operatively was minimal. Alcoholic hepatitis is therefore unlikely.

(2) Biliary obstruction (either intra-hepatic or extra-hepatic) should be excluded. Laparotomy was normal, and it is unlikely that there was a significant extra-hepatic cause for the obstruction (such as carcinoma or gallstones). As the liver function tests returned to normal by the time of discharge from hospital it is unlikely that intra-hepatic cholestasis is the basis for the further abnormalities. The early episode of cholestatic jaundice could be explained by 'benign post-operative intrahepatic cholestasis' which is a condition of multi-factorial aetiology including trauma, hypotension, sepsis and transfusion.

(3) Halothane. This causes hypersensitivity hepatitis which has a delayed onset following the anaesthetic and is associated with multiple exposure to halothane. The initial abnormality of liver function tests probably occurred too early following exposure and

presented a picture of cholestasis rather than hepatitis. The onset of hepatitis caused by halothane as late as 2 weeks after exposure is rare and it is extremely rare for this hepatitis to become chronic.

(4) Hepatitis B. Since donor blood is screened for hepatitis B antigen it is unlikely (but possible) that the hepatitis was caused by this agent. The incubation period is usually between 3 and 4 months and the hepatitis in this case, therefore, developed rather early for it to be the result of infection with hepatitis B virus.

(5) Hepatitis A. This is not associated with post-transfusion hepatitis. There is no documented evidence of chronic hepatitis following hepatitis A exposure and hepatitis A at the age of 62 years would be unlikely.

(6) Epstein–Barr or cytomegalovirus infection. Both may cause hepatitis but there is little evidence that they are responsible for post-transfusion hepatitis in immunocompetant patients.

(7) Non-A, non-B hepatitis. This has an incubation period of about 7 weeks, i.e. between the incubation period of hepatitis A (3–4 weeks) and of hepatitis B (3–4 months). It is now thought to be the commonest cause of post-transfusion hepatitis. It is frequently asymptomatic and anicteric and may produce chronic disease. The histology is similar to that of chronic active hepatitis with piecemeal necrosis and there may be progression to cirrhosis, although the chronic active hepatitis tends to have a more benign course than that caused by hepatitis B.

(1) Investigations which should be performed include:
   (a) Hepatitis B surface antigen and antibody
   (b) Percutaneous liver biopsy
   (c) Epstein Barr and cytomegalovirus titres
(2) The most likely diagnosis is non-A, non-B post-transfusion hepatitis.

Answers:

This man has evidence of cirrhosis (liver scan appearance, low plasma albumin, and splenomegaly) which was probably present at the age of 11 years. As a homosexual he may well be a carrier of hepatitis B but the history suggests a recent acute hepatitis. It is very unlikely that hepatitis B was present at the age of 11 years but it is more likely to have been acquired recently during homosexual activities. Carriage of the antigen is likely to persist in these homosexual patients and be highly transmissible particularly in the presence of e antigen. Another cause for cirrhosis must be sought.

Neonatal jaundice leading to cirrhosis is most likely to be due to alpha-1-antitrypsin deficiency. Patients with 'neonatal hepatitis' tend to recover and do not progress to cirrhosis. Alpha-1-antitrypsin deficiency is second only to extrahepatic biliary atresia as a cause of cholestatic jaundice in infancy. Patients in the latter group remain jaundiced and soon die.

Alpha-1-antitrypsin is synthesized in hepatocytes. Deficiency is inherited and usually associated with phenotype ZZ. In these patients the hepatocytes contain characteristic globules thought to be the result of accumulation of the precursor of alpha-1-antitrypsin which cannot be released from the cell. The mechanism of liver damage is unknown.

(1) Acute hepatitis B is the most likely cause of his present illness. An intercurrent infection which caused decompensation of cirrhosis is also possible.

(2) Diagnostic investigations are:
   (a) percutaneous liver biopsy. This may show inclusion bodies of alpha-1-antitrypsin precursor. Ground glass cells associated with hepatitis B may develop later.
   (b) plasma protein electrophoresis to show alpha-1-antitrypsin deficiency.

A24

Answers:

(1) The most likely diagnosis is *Strep. milleri* liver abscess. Liver abscess should be considered in cases of pyrexia of unknown origin where sepsis is a likely cause, particularly when *Strep. milleri* is isolated from the blood: a recent review of the bacteriology of liver abscess showed that 13 out of 16 cases were caused by this organism[1]. Liver abscess is associated with a high mortality (approximately 50%) and this is the result of late diagnosis (often at necropsy).

The causative organisms may be Gram-negative Enterobacteriaceae (from the gut) but with improved methods of culture, anaerobes – such as Bacteroides – have been isolated, and more recently *Strep. milleri* has been distinguished from these. This distinction is important as *Strep. milleri* is resistant to metronidazole and sensitive to penicillin. Blood cultures will be positive in fewer than 40% of patients with a liver abscess, but culture of aspirate from the abscess is much more helpful (approximately 80% positive).

Liver abscess may be secondary to ruptured intra-abdominal viscus, inflammatory bowel disease, bacterial cholangitis or cancer, but in about 50% of cases no underlying cause is apparent. Abscesses are more common in the right lobe of the liver, and this is thought to be a function of the drainage of blood from the right colon.

Other diagnoses which should be considered in this case include amoebic liver abscess (in view of the previous history of dysentery when in the Far East), which may have flared up when the patient was treated with steroids, and tuberculosis, which should be considered in elderly patients with abnormal chest radiographs who are also taking steroids.

(2) (a) Probably the best investigation to determine the size, site and number of hepatic abscesses is ultrasonography. This may also demonstrate biliary tract disease. Depending on available facilities, technetium liver scan, gallium scan, computed tomography or hepatic arteriography will all give useful information. Aspiration of pus under ultrasonographic or CT guidance may give accurate bacteriological diagnosis (particularly when blood cultures are negative).

    (b) Serological test for amoebiasis (positive in over 90% of patients with amoebic liver abscesses).

   (c) Sigmoidoscopy and biopsy.
(3) (a) As the bacteriological diagnosis is known (*Strep. milleri*), intravenous benzylpenicillin is the treatment of choice; otherwise, a combination of penicillin, gentamicin and metronidazole would be suitable.
   (b) If the abscess is large and does not rapidly reduce in size with antibiotic therapy, it should be drained surgically; this is probably best done percutaneously with ultrasound guidance. Installation of antibiotics directly into the abscess cavity is thought to be unnecessary.

Liver abscess is a rare condition, but should be suspected in a febrile patient with an enlarged, tender liver and elevated alkaline phosphatase, an erythrocyte sedimentation rate greater than 100 mm/h, normochromic normocytic anaemia and reduction in plasma albumin. The presence of jaundice suggests multicentric abscesses and is thus a bad prognostic sign.

Reference

Moore-Gillan, J. C., Eykyn, S. J. and Phillips, I. (1981). Microbiology of pyogenic liver abscess. *Br. Med. J.*, 2, 819

Further Reading

Leading article (1980). Pyogenic liver abscess. *Br. Med. J.*, 1, 1155–6
Perera, M. R., Kirk, A. and Noone, P. (1980). Presentation, diagnosis and management of liver abscess. *Lancet*, 2, 629

Answers: A25

(1) This is shock resistant to volume replacement with a clotting abnormality in a young, previously healthy man with a 48 hour history of non-specific illness. The most likely diagnosis is septicaemia.
(2) (a) There is a family history of anaemia, and the patient had an abdominal scar. He may have had a splenectomy. Such individuals are particularly susceptible to pneumococcal septicaemia. (Splenectomy following trauma may result in seeding of splenic tissue in the peritoneal cavity and this reduces the susceptibility.)

    (b) Septicaemia complicating leukaemia.

    (c) Meningococcal septicaemia. This may cause shock and a purpuric skin rash in a young healthy person. It is likely, however, that the lumbar puncture would have shown evidence of meningitis.

    (d) Staphylococcal septicaemia complicating influenza.

    (e) Septicaemia complicating an aplastic process, possibly drug-induced.

    (f) Snake bite may produce a similar picture, but in the UK adder bites have only local effects on adults.

(3) (a) Disseminated intravascular coagulation.

    (b) Large numbers of bacteria in the blood metabolize glucose. This probably happens in the sample tube awaiting analysis (rather than *in vivo*) as suggested by the normal cerebrospinal fluid glucose concentration.

    (c) Sequestration of granulocytes in the lung. In experimental models of pneumococcal septicaemia massive numbers of granulocytes and platelets lodge in the pulmonary capillaries with extensive fibrin deposition leading to ventilation–perfusion abnormalities. This may explain the patient's tachypnoea.

    (d) The syndrome of inappropriate secretion of antidiuretic hormone (SIADH).

A26 Answers:

This is a middle-aged man with a 4 month history of weakness, diffuse pain and weight loss who has a cough fracture. He has proximal myopathy and increased bowel sounds with diffuse musculo-skeletal pain, anaemia, raised alkaline phosphatase and low plasma phosphate. The differential diagnosis must include carcinomatosis (the bronchus being the most likely primary), hyperthyroidism, polymyalgia rheumatica and osteomalacia. Of these osteomalacia is the most likely because of the clinical picture, the low plasma phosphate and evidence of secondary hyperparathyroidism (erosion of the distal ends of the clavicles).

Investigations should be directed towards limiting the differential diagnosis and, in the case of osteomalacia, establishing its cause. A distended abdomen with increased bowel sounds and macrocytic

anaemia suggests malabsorption as the cause of the osteomalacia.
Investigations should include:

(1) ^{99}Tc pyrophosphate bone scan – this may show symmetrical discrete areas of increased uptake suggestive of metabolic bone disease or may suggest secondary carcinoma. The investigation may be followed by limited radiological skeletal survey directed by the 'hot spots'. If Looser's zones are present this is diagnostic of osteomalacia.

(2) Bone biopsy. In the absence of Looser's zones this may be used to diagnose osteomalacia.

(3) Three-day faecal fat estimation.

(4) Serum B_{12} and red cell folate estimation.

(5) Barium follow-through.

(6) *Per oral* (Crosby capsule) jejunal biopsy.

(7) Sputum cytology.

(8) Thyroid function tests.

Section 2
SLIDE INTERPRETATION

Q1

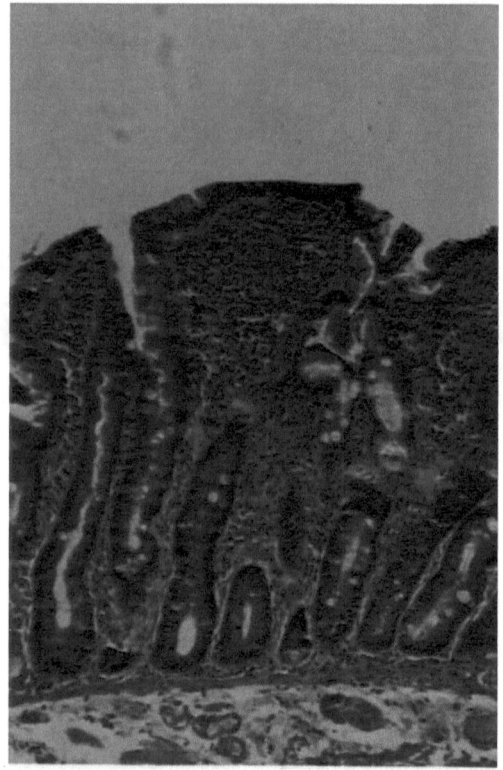

This is a biopsy specimen viewed under a low-power microscope lens.

(1) What abnormalities do you see?

(2) What biochemical abnormalities would you expect to find in the venous blood?

(3) How would you confirm your diagnosis?

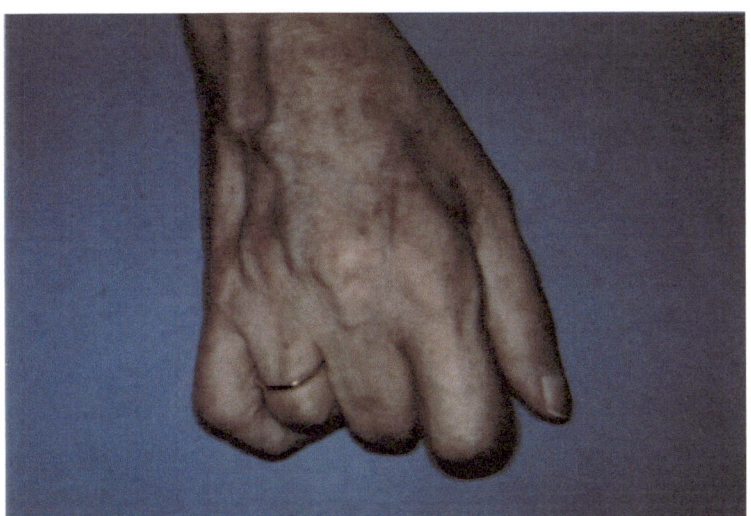

Q2

(1) What abnormality do you see in the hand of this lady whose fist is lightly clenched?
(2) What 3 conditions may be associated with this abnormality?

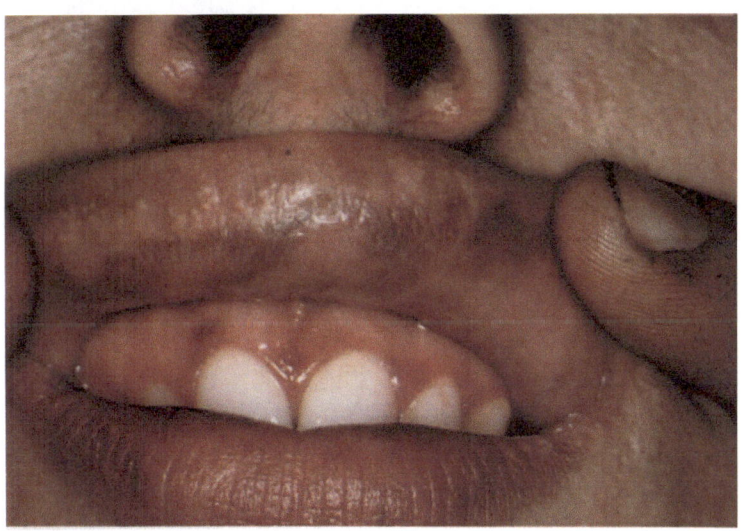

Q3

(1) Describe the abnormality.
(2) What is the likely cause?

Q4

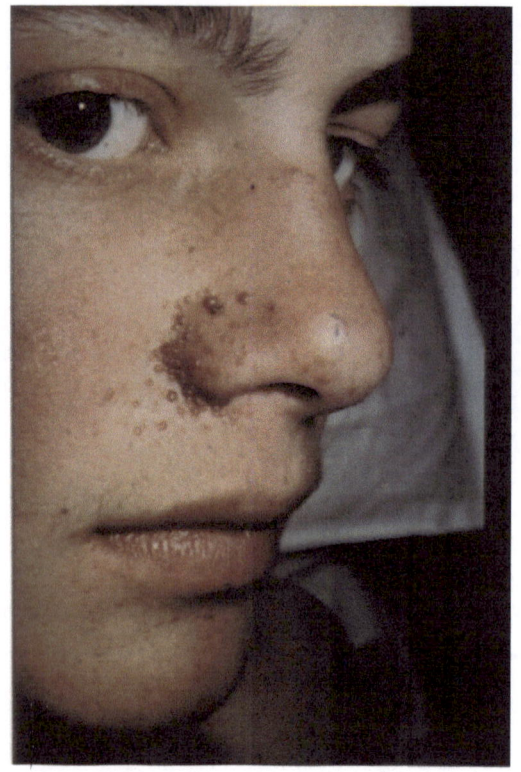

This is a 9-year-old boy who is mentally retarded.

(1) What 2 abnormalities are shown?

(2) How are they related?

(3) What other skin lesions may be present?

Q5

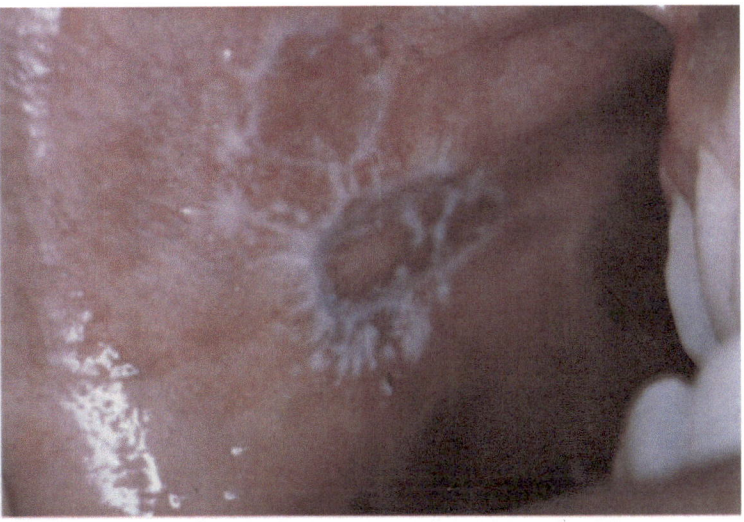

(1) What is this condition?
(2) Describe the characteristic features which enable you to make the diagnosis.
(3) On what areas of the body are the other lesions of this condition commonly found?

Q6

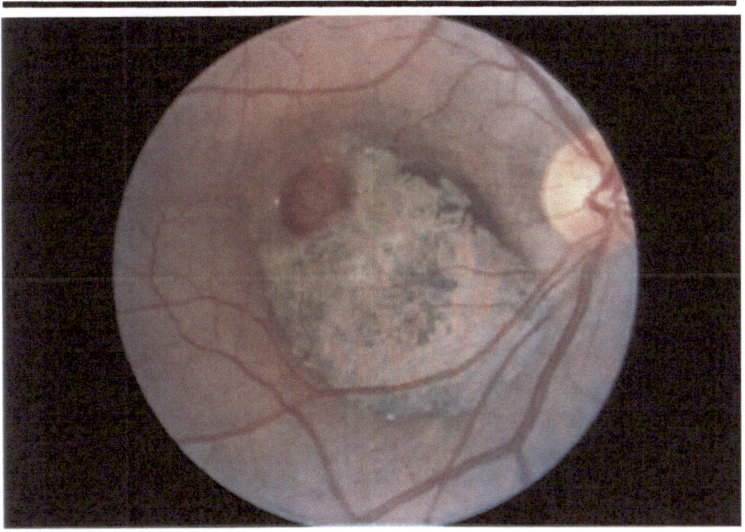

What is this fundal appearance?

Q7

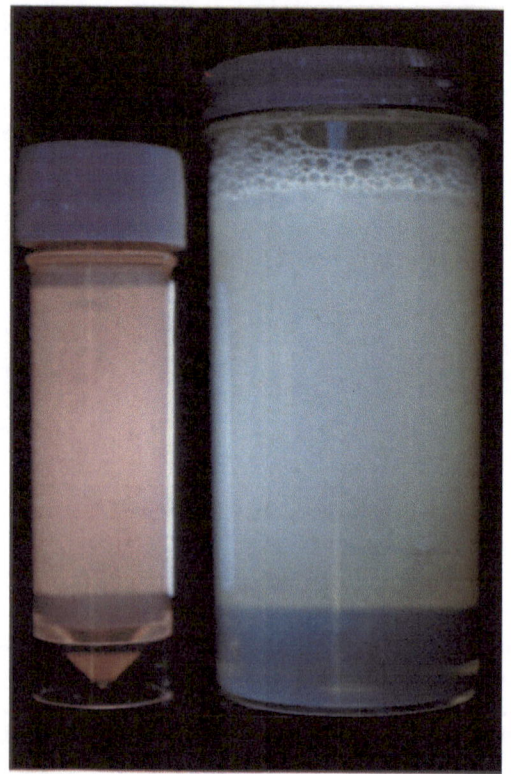

A 55-year-old male publican presented with a rash on his face and forearms which was considerably improved in the cold weather. The picture is of a specimen of his urine beside a specimen of normal urine.
(1) What procedure has been performed to account for the difference between the 2 specimens?
(2) What is the diagnosis?
(3) Of what other symptoms may the patient complain?
(4) What treatment would you consider?

Q8

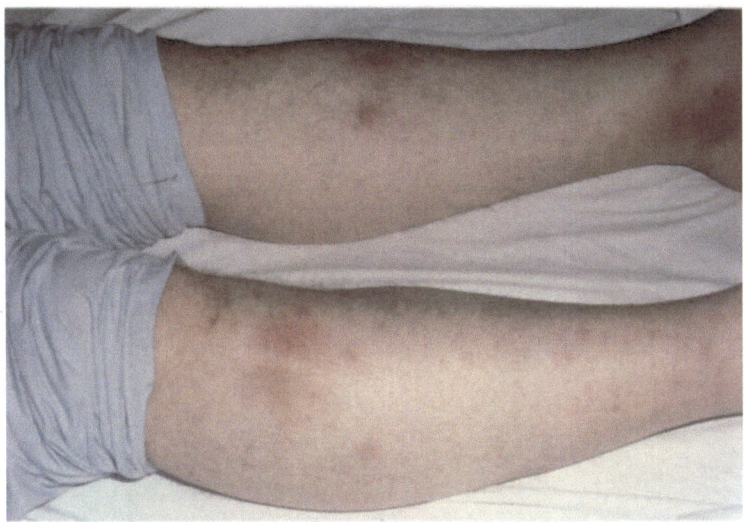

This slide shows the lower legs of a 26-year-old man presenting with arthralgia of the knees and ankles, pyrexia and these tender skin lesions.

(1) What is the diagnosis?
(2) What are the causes of this condition?

Q9

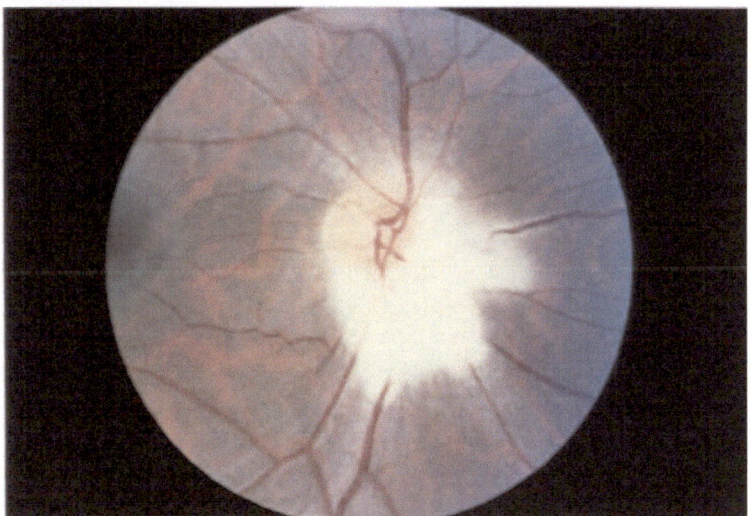

What is this fundal appearance due to?

Q10

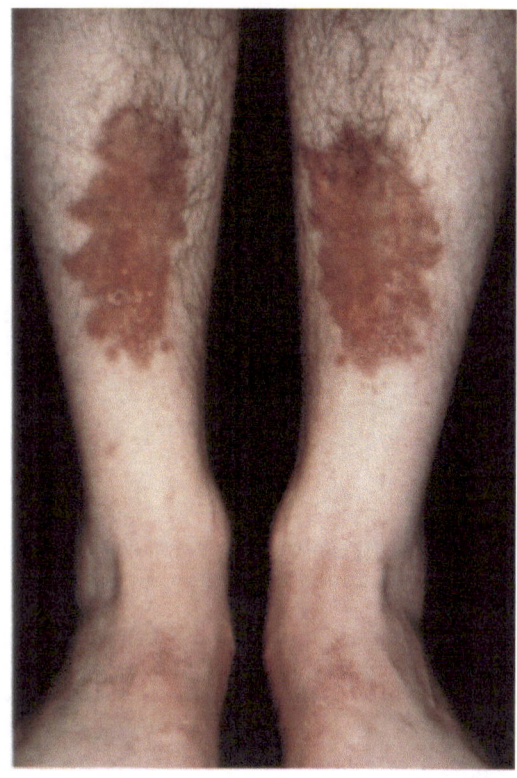

(1) What is this condition?
(2) What is its relationship to underlying systemic disease?

Q11

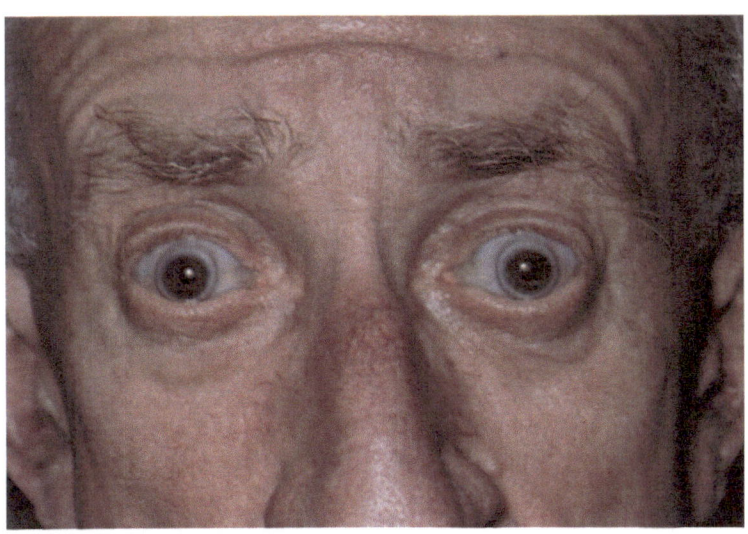

(1) What is the diagnosis?
(2) What is the commonest mode of inheritance?
(3) What are the associated abnormalities?

Q12

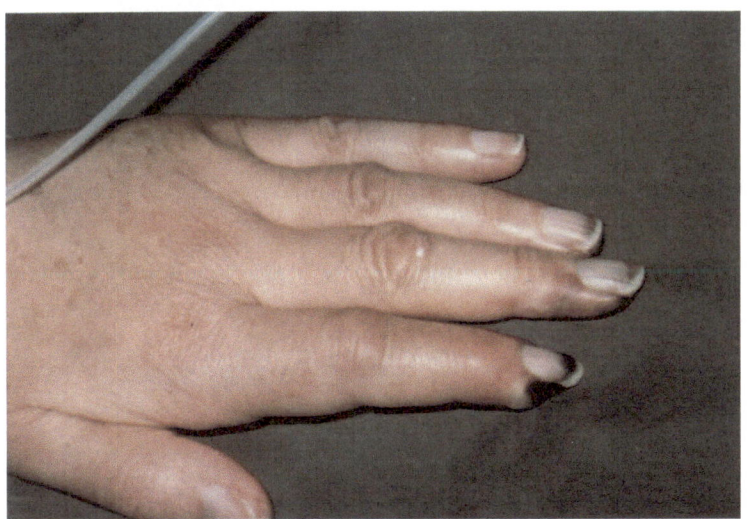

(1) Describe the appearance of these hands.
(2) Suggest possible causes for this appearance.

Q13

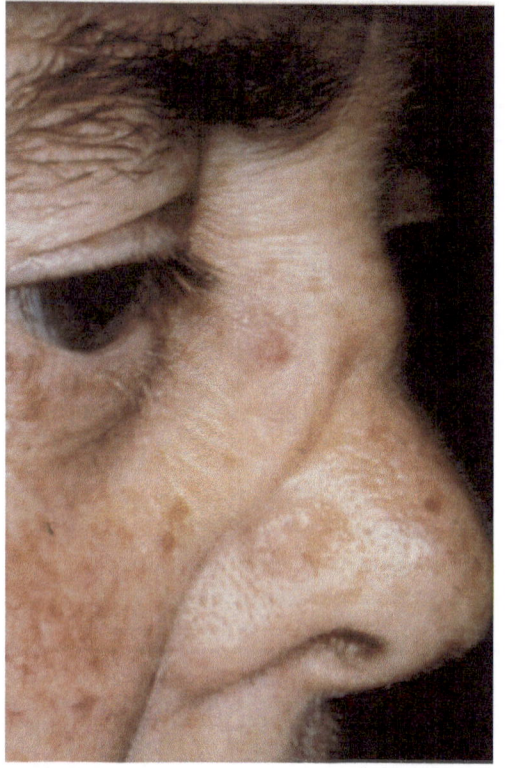

This is a 55-year-old lady whose facial profile was normal until 5 years ago. There is no history of trauma.

(1) What is the diagnosis?

(2) What other features may be present?

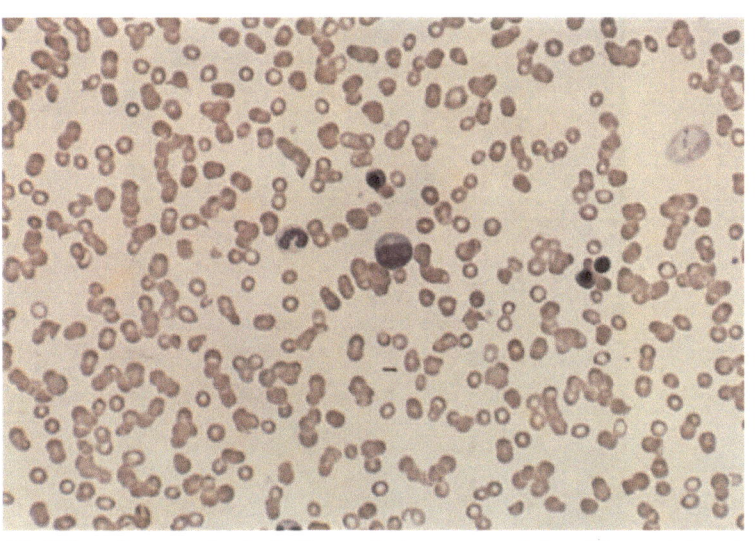

Q14

(1) What haematological diagnosis is suggested by this peripheral blood film?
(2) List the causes of this abnormality.

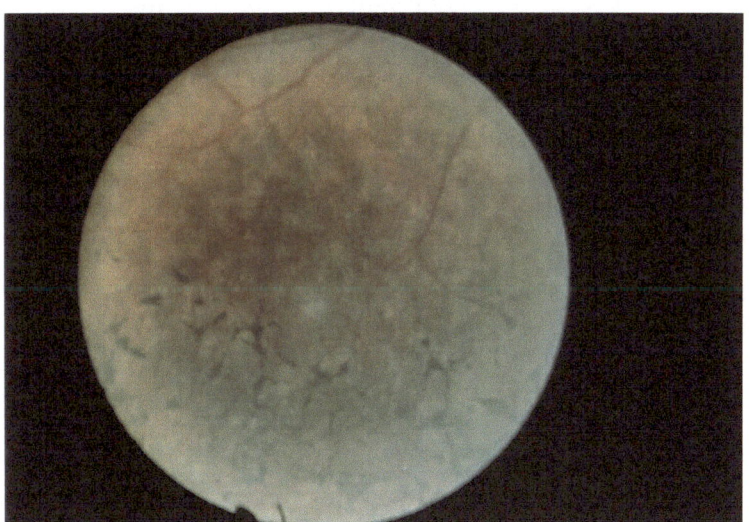

Q15

(1) What retinal abnormality is shown?
(2) With which conditions is it associated?

Q16

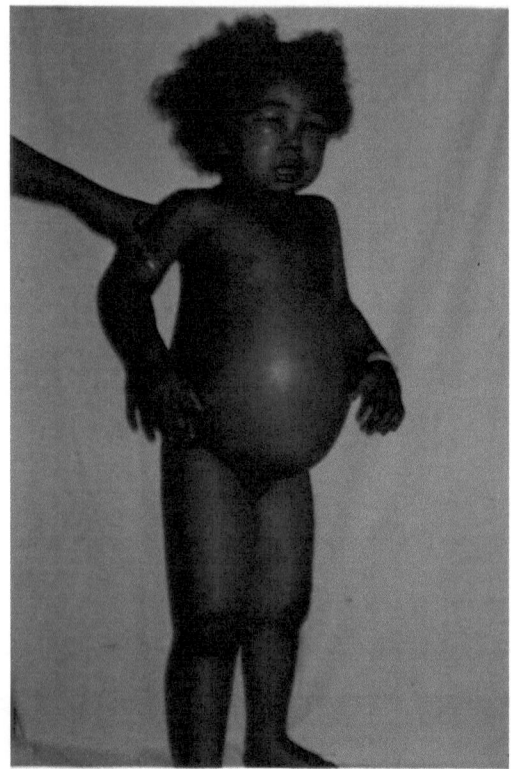

(1) What is the likely cause of this appearance?

(2) Give 3 pathological entities which may form the basis of this appearance.

Q17

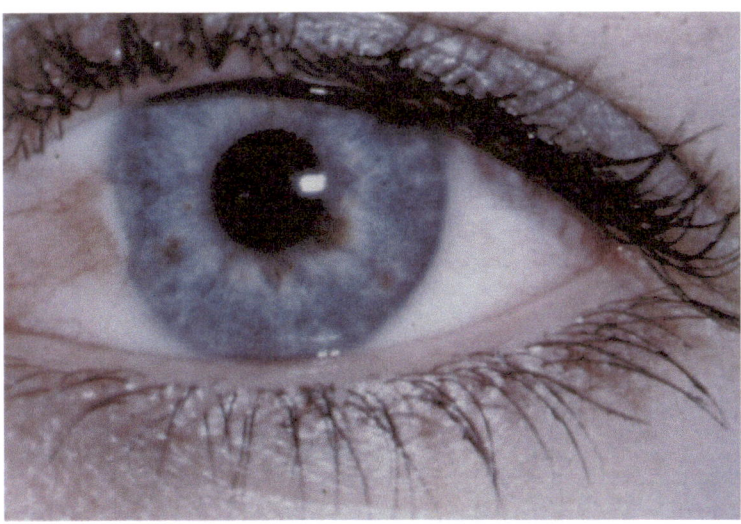

(1) What abnormality is shown?
(2) What symptoms are likely to be associated?
(3) Describe the likely environment from which this patient came.

Q18

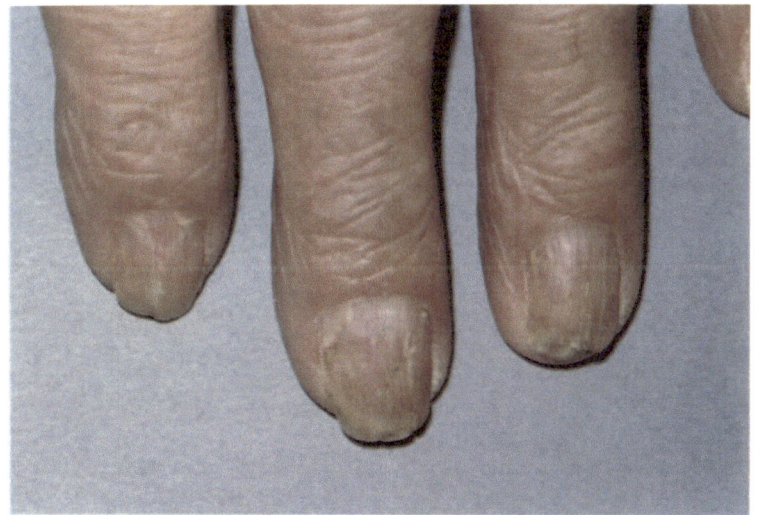

(1) What condition has caused these nail changes?
(2) What other features may be present?

Q19

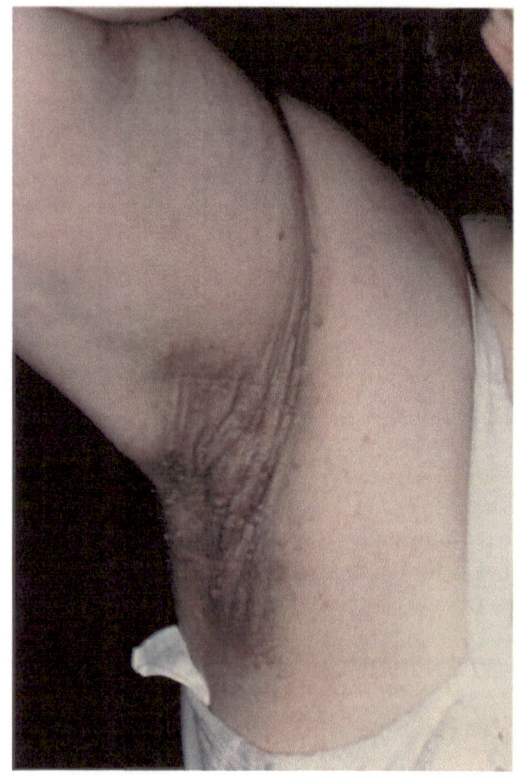

(1) What is this lesion?
(2) With what conditions may it be associated?

Q20

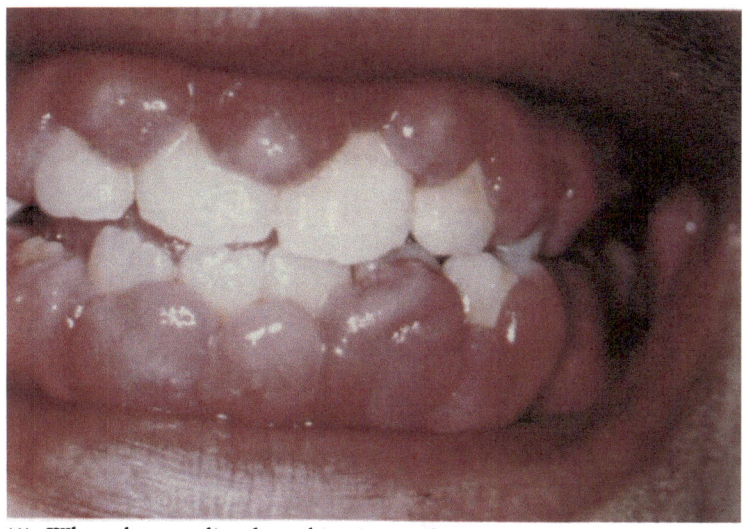

(1) What abnormality does this picture demonstrate?
(2) Give 3 causes of such an appearance.

Q21

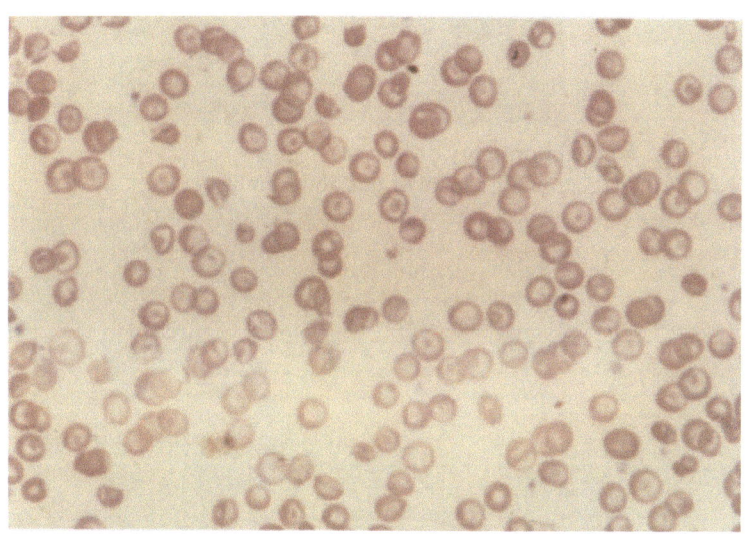

(1) Describe the haematological abnormality on this peripheral blood film.
(2) What conditions are associated with this?

Q22

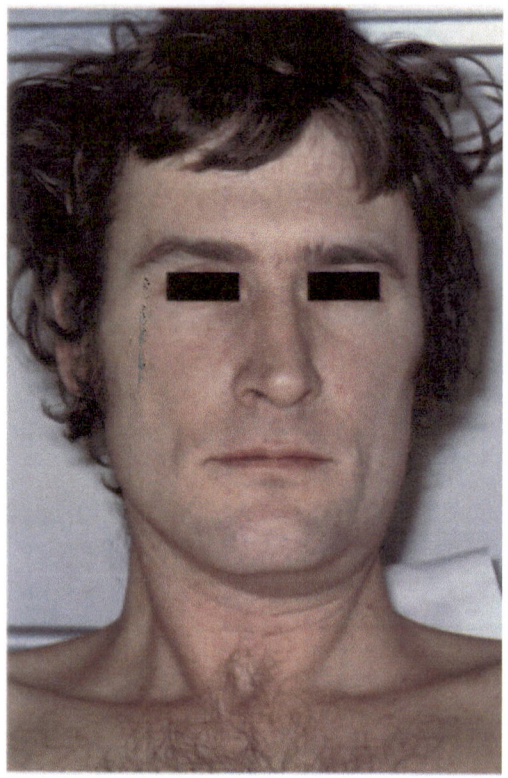

(1) What abnormality do you see?
(2) List 5 possible causes of this abnormality.

Q23

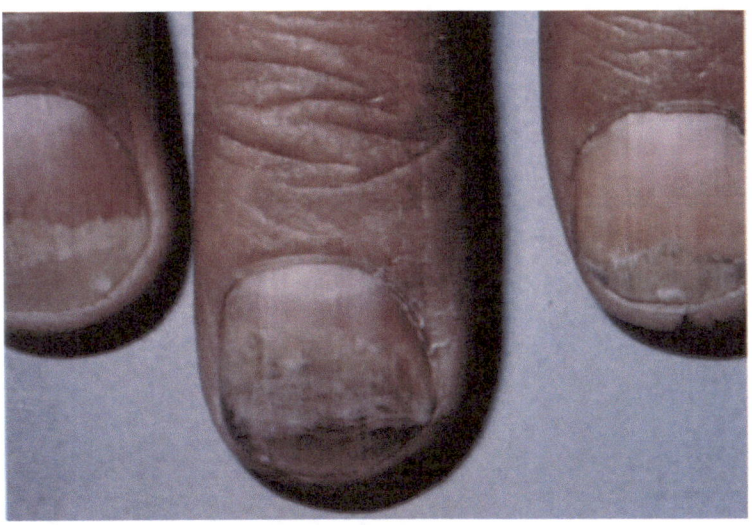

(1) What is the nail abnormality shown?
(2) What are the causes of this abnormality?

Q24

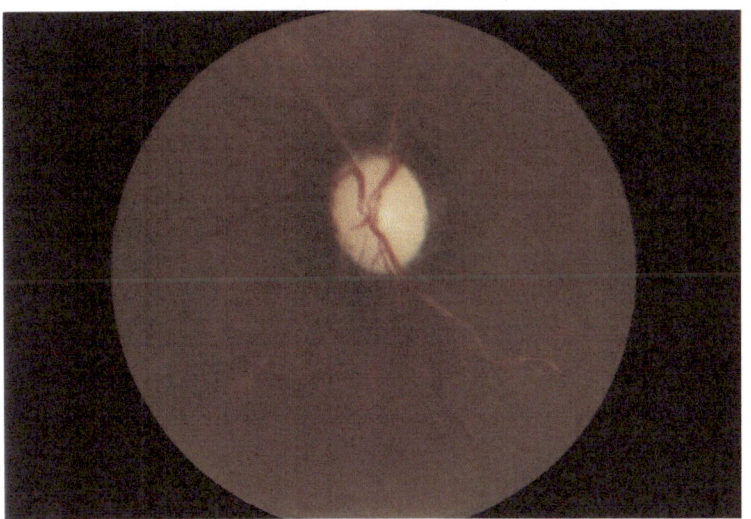

(1) Describe the appearance of this retina.
(2) Give 2 possible causes.

Q25

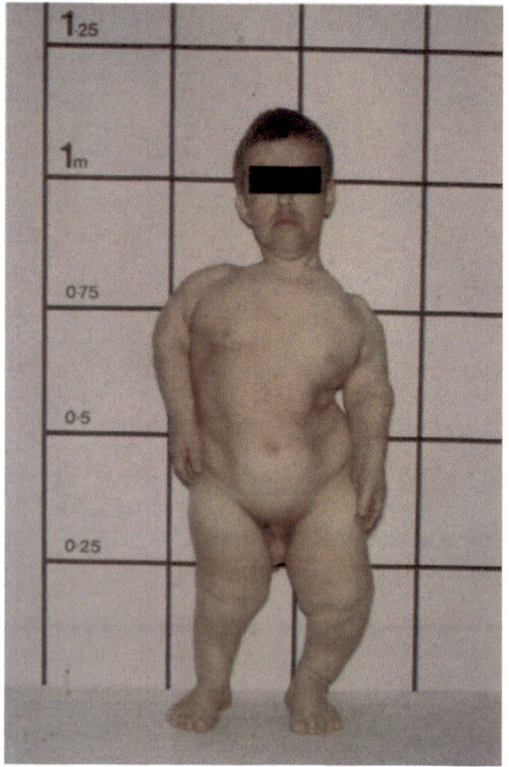

This is a 40-year-old man of normal intelligence, taking no regular medication, with normal plasma biochemistry and no radiologically demonstrable fractures.

(1) What is the diagnosis?

(2) Document the features that support this diagnosis.

Q26

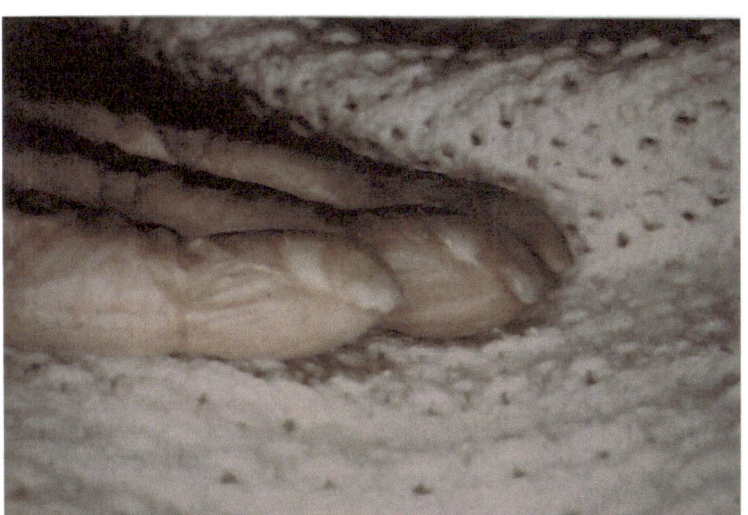

(1) Document the 2 abnormalities shown in this picture.
(2) What is the diagnosis?

Q27

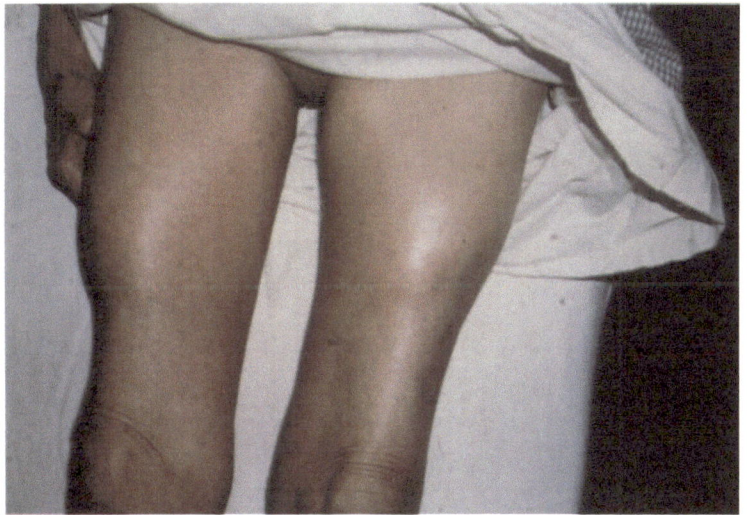

(1) What is the most likely diagnosis?
(2) Name 4 features which may be associated with this.

Q28

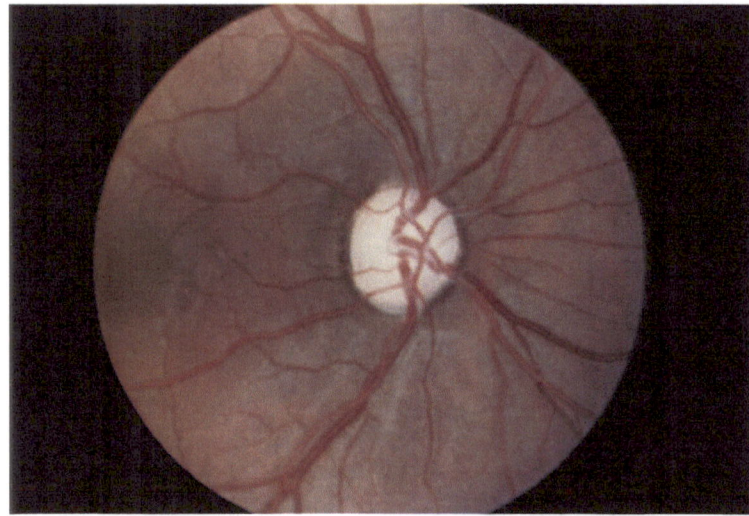

(1) Describe the appearance of this optic fundus and give the diagnosis.
(2) With what conditions is this finding associated?

Q29

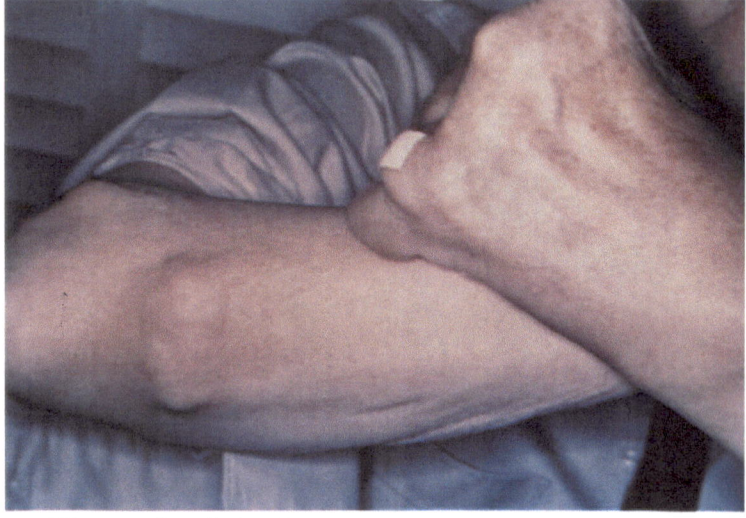

(1) What are these lesions?
(2) Discuss their relationship to underlying systemic disease.

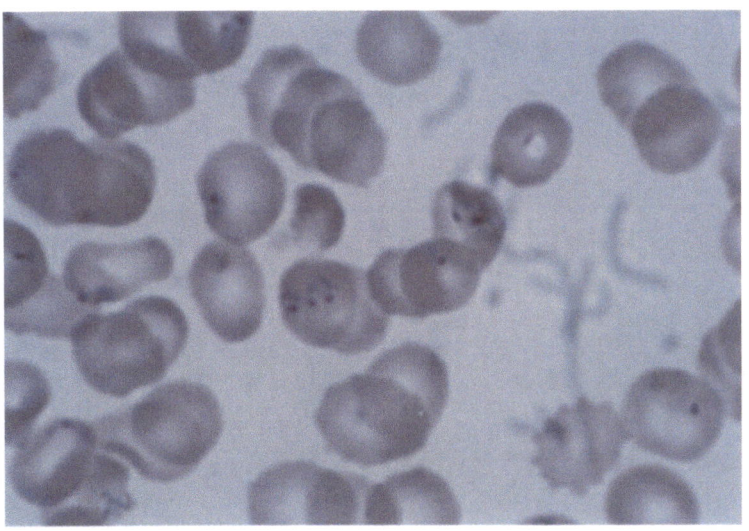

Q30

(1) What abnormality is seen in this peripheral blood film?
(2) What is the likely aetiology of the abnormality?

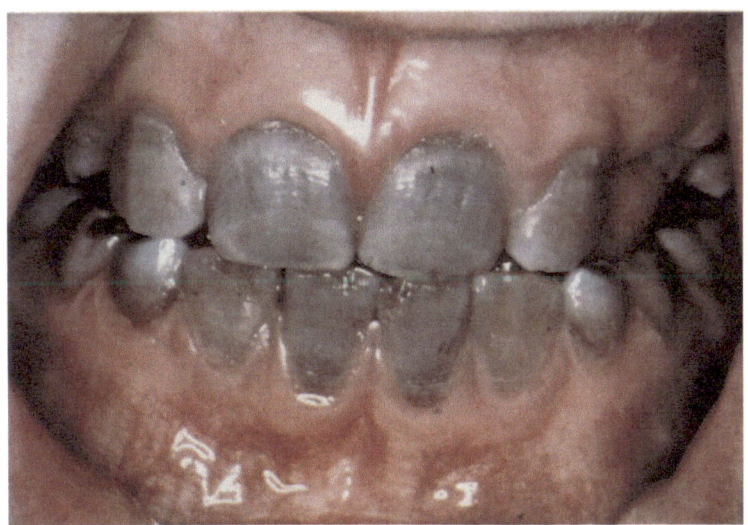

Q31

(1) What is the most likely cause of this appearance?
(2) Give 3 other possible but less likely diagnoses.

Q32

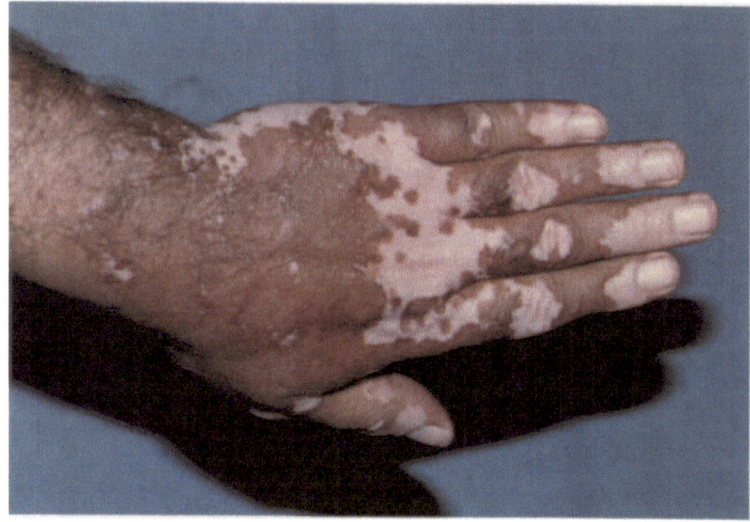

(1) What is this condition?

(2) With what disorders is it associated?

AIDS FOR X-RAY INTERPRETATION

Initial Inspection of an X-ray

(1) Read the name label
  - this gives an idea of the patient's sex (if female note if both breast shadows are visible) which may also influence one's differential diagnosis.
  - may also indicate nationality.
  - may give name of the hospital and hence the country or area of origin.

(2) Look for 'left' or 'right' label.

(3) Read all the other writing on the film
  - the diagnosis may be written.
  - IVU - control time, etc.
  - Date - sequential films.

(4) Note how the film is taken
  - PA, AP, degree of inspiration. Erect or supine.

(5) Have a system for interpreting each film

(a) *Where a lesion is obvious at initial inspection of the film* - comment on the abnormality before considering the rest of the film.

  (i) Describe the abnormality - do not suggest an immediate diagnosis as it may be wrong. Describe site, size, character of the edge, presence or absence of calcification and any abnormalities in the surrounding lung.

  (ii) Consider the rest of the film. If any other abnormalities are seen during this search then each of these should be described in turn.

  (iii) Gather the abnormalities and any clinical information together and from this make your differential diagnosis, giving the most likely diagnosis first.

(b) *Where initial viewing of the film shows no abnormality*
Say that you cannot see an abnormality and proceed to a system by system analysis of the film.

Interpretation of the Chest Radiograph

A. *The Heart*

(1) Size. The cardiothoracic ratio is not a good guide to cardiac size because in the elderly the thoracic cavity contracts. The upper limit of the transverse diameter of the heart is: Men 16 cm, Women 15 cm. A variation of cardiac diameter between films of up to 1 cm is allowed for the difference in size between systole and diastole.

(2) Shape. This is variable and only enlargement of the left atrium can be confidently diagnosed. A left ventricular aneurysm may result in an abnormal left heart border.

(3) Calcification.

- aortic and mitral valves often calcify when diseased, as may the ring surrounding the mitral valve.
- pericardium, secondary to tuberculosis or haemorrhage.
- heart muscle, post-infarction.
- thrombus in an aneurysm of the left ventricle or in the left atrium.
- cardiac tumours (rare).
- coronary vessels (of no prognostic value).

B. *Hila*

Hilar shadows represent the pulmonary arteries and the left is normally higher than the right.

(1) calcification
- TB adenitis (common)
- histoplasmosis
- eggshell - sarcoidosis
          asbestosis
          berylliosis

(2) enlargement
- unilateral
    - cancer
    - node enlargement
    - pulmonary stenosis (left)
- bilateral
    - sarcoidosis
    - lymphoma - often asymmetrical and may also involve the paratracheal nodes

- leukaemia
- infectious mononucleosis
- chronic airflow obstruction
- asthma
- cystic fibrosis
- left ventricular failure - large hilar shadows with fluffy edges due to peri-hilar oedema.

(3) position
- elevated due to
  - bilateral apical fibrosis in tuberculosis
  - upper lobe resection
  - radiation therapy
  - ankylosing spondylitis
  - extrinsic allergic alveolitis
  - pneumoconiosis
- depressed due to
  - collapse of the lower lobes
  - radiation damage to the bases
  - surgical resection.

C. *Mediastinum*

(1) Aorta
   enlarged
   - aneurysm (Marfan's or syphilitic in the ascending part)
   - post-stenotic dilatation
   - dissection
   calcified
   - atheromatous aortic knuckle.

(2) Oesophagus - not normally seen but if visible, it is dilated and may have a fluid level
   - achalasia
   - obstruction - carcinoma or stenosis
   - large incarcerated hiatus hernia
   - pharyngeal pouch
   - Chagas disease (rare)
   - scleroderma (note no fluid level seen on erect film).

(3) Wide
   - aortic dissection
   - nodes
   - tumour
   - mediastinitis.

(4) Free air (emphysema)
- asthma
- ruptured oesophagus
- pregnancy
- weight lifting
- deep sea diving.

D. *Lungs*

Be aware of variations in the normal anatomy (see Figure 1).

(1) consolidation. This is a radiological term indicating white shadowing, and the description should include site, i.e. lobe, segment or whole lung. Causes:
- infection - air bronchogram usually seen
- obstruction - no air bronchogram present and anatomically lobar or segmental consolidation
- infarction
- aspiration
- contusion
- intrapulmonary haemorrhage
- pulmonary oedema (alveolar)
- radiotherapy.

(2) collapse. Rarely present without consolidation but may be seen with bronchial obstruction (see Figure 2 (a–f)).

(3) opacities
- primary or secondary tumours
- granulomata
- hamartoma (calcified 'popcorn')
- A–V malformation
- pulmonary infarct
- pulmonary abscess
- pseudotumours due to pleural fluid in fissures
- hydatid
- haematoma (post-trauma).

(4) cavitating lesions
- primary or secondary tumours
- abscess
- granulomata (Wegener's, Caplan's syndrome, rheumatoid)
- infarction.

ACCESSORY FISSURES

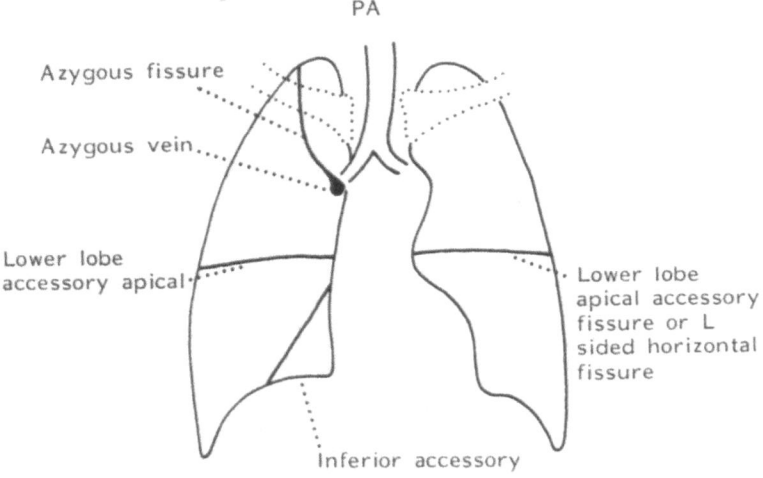

PA

Azygous fissure

Azygous vein

Lower lobe
accessory apical

Lower lobe
apical accessory
fissure or L
sided horizontal
fissure

Inferior accessory

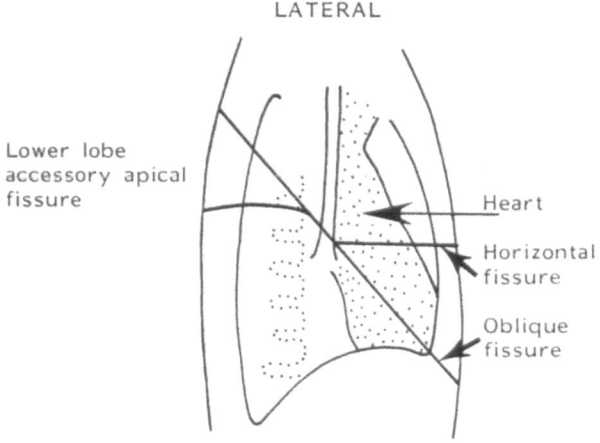

LATERAL

Lower lobe
accessory apical
fissure

Heart

Horizontal
fissure

Oblique
fissure

Figure 1

89

PATTERNS OF LOBAR COLLAPSE

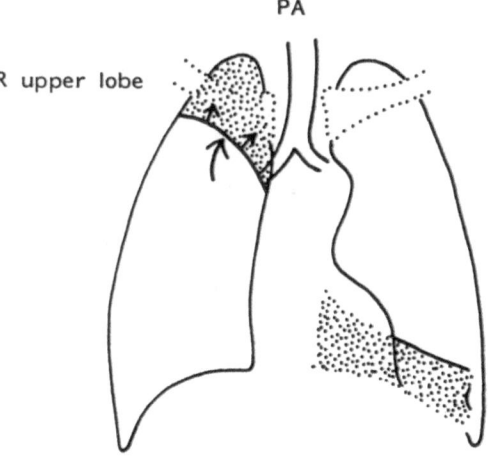

NB: L hemidiaphragm
disappears

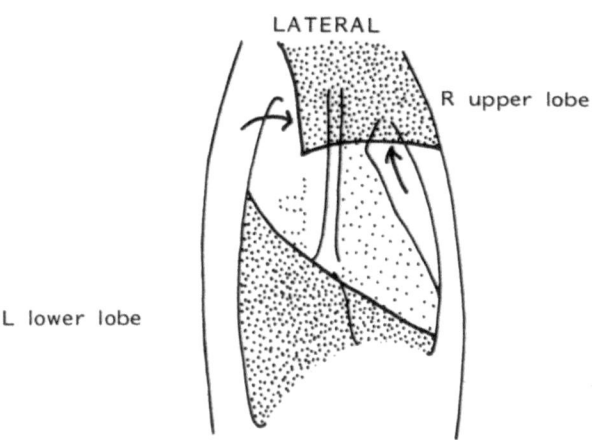

Figure 2,a,b

PA

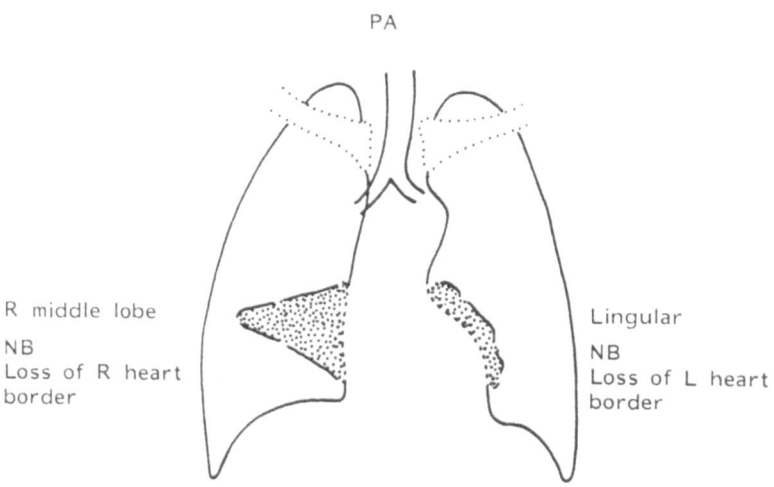

R middle lobe

NB
Loss of R heart
border

Lingular

NB
Loss of L heart
border

LATERAL

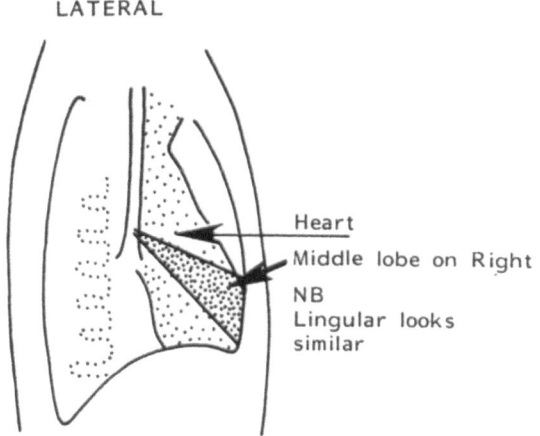

Heart

Middle lobe on Right

NB
Lingular looks
similar

Figure 2,c,d

P.A.

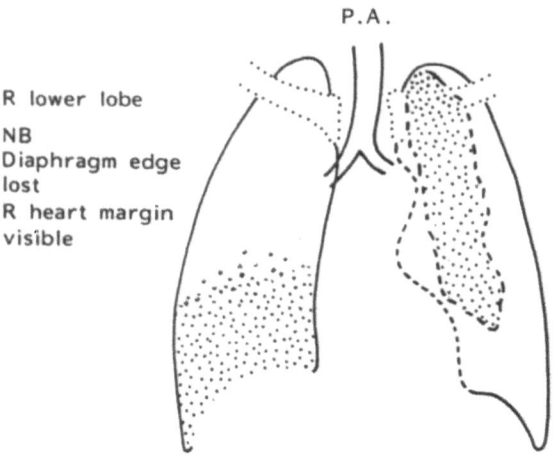

R lower lobe

NB
Diaphragm edge
lost
R heart margin
visible

L upper lobe
vague upper and
middle zone density.
L heart border lost.
NB
Lingular bronchus
comes off upper
bronchus division

LATERAL

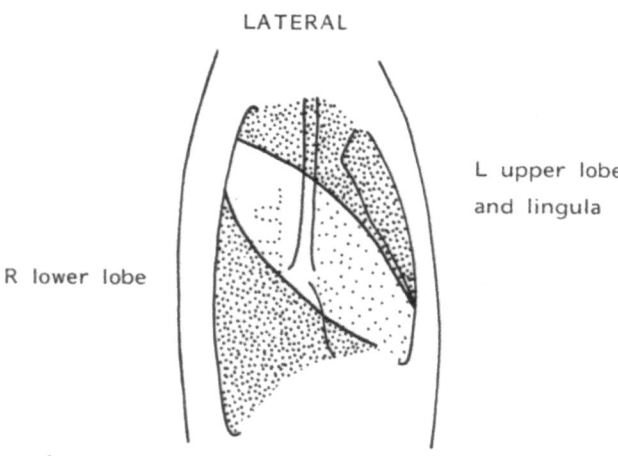

R lower lobe

L upper lobe
and lingula

Figure 2,e,f

(5) septal lines (Kerley's B lines) due to fluid in or thickening of the inter-lobular septa.
  - LV failure
  - mitral stenosis
  - fluid overload
  - renal failure
  - toxic gases
  - blast injury
  - raised intra-cranial pressure
  - industrial diseases (pneumoconiosis)
  - sarcoidosis
  - Hodgkin's
  - lymphangitis carcinomatosa.

E. *Pleura*

  (1) fluid
  - collects in dependent regions and will vary with the position of the patient
  - appears to creep up the chest wall
  - may be loculated in a fissure or against the chest wall
  - may be sub-pulmonary, and the diaphragm appears elevated
  - up to 400 ml behind the diaphragmatic dome may be invisible on PA erect film
  - in children may lie along the lateral chest wall only, even on an erect film
  - pus, blood, lymph, transudates and exudates all appear identical on an X-ray and cannot be distinguished by any simple radiographic means.

  (2) thickening
  - post-infection (tuberculosis often in the apical region)
  - asbestos exposure (usually bilateral against the lateral chest wall)
  - primary or secondary pleural tumours
  - reaction to adjacent bone lesions.

  (3) calcification
  - tuberculosis

- asbestos plaques (often seen over the diaphragmatic surfaces)
- mica exposure.

F. *Bones*

    (1) ribs

        - fractures due to trauma or osteomalacia

        - secondary deposits especially in myeloma

        - notching.

    (2) clavicles

        - erosion of the lateral ends (hyperparathyroidism).

G. *Soft Tissues*

Primary skin lesions may be projected over the lungs and appear as pulmonary opacities.

Hypertranslucency of a lung field (having excluded patient rotation) is usually due to soft tissue abnormalities, e.g. absent pectoral muscle following mastectomy, poliomyelitis, Macleod's syndrome.

H. *The sub-phrenic area*

This is also included on a chest film and should routinely be inspected for:

    - the stomach gas bubble

    - fluid levels beneath the diaphragm (sub-phrenic abscess)

    - calcium below the diaphragm.

Interpretation of the Abdominal Radiograph

Most information is to be found on a supine *not* erect film
Look at *all* areas and then concentrate on the following.

A. *Gas Patterns*

    (1) *Bowel gas*

        - stomach gas is seen in the left upper quadrant (a gas fluid level in the erect film and band shadows of the gastric rugae in supine view). Right sided gastric shadow suggests *situs inversus*.

        - duodenum often contains air and a fluid level

        - small bowel tends to be centrally placed and when

distended may show complete transverse bands (*valvulae conniventes*). These are close together (<5 mm)
- large bowel tends to be peripheral with haustra usually visible (incomplete bands across colonic gas shadow >1 cm apart).
- large bowel should not be larger than 5 cm diameter and small bowel 3.5 cm diameter.
- fluid levels - only useful on erect film and in conjunction with dilatation of the bowel. In the small intestine more than 2 fluid levels greater than 2.5 cm in length suggest obstruction or ileus.

(2) *Bowel wall gas*
- necrosis, e.g. ischaemic or necrotizing enterocolitis
- pneumatosis cystoides intestinalis.

(3) *Abdominal gas*
- if both sides of the bowel wall can be seen when no loops are lying adjacent, free abdominal gas is present. It will collect centrally within the abdomen on a supine film and can be confirmed on an erect film.
- is a normal finding within 7 days of laparotomy, but otherwise suggests perforation of a gas-containing viscus. Large amounts suggest perforation of the large bowel (e.g. caecum).

(4) *Gas elsewhere*
  (a) in the biliary tree
    - gallstone ileus (in association with small bowel obstruction)
    - post-surgery
    - recent passage of gallstone.
  (b) in portal vein suggesting portal pyaemia with gas-forming organism.
  (c) within the kidneys or bladder - gas forming infection possibly associated with diabetes mellitus.
  (d) psoas or retro-peritoneum
    - infection
    - trauma
  (e) small gas bubbles in groups - abscess, for example in the bed of the pancreas in severe pancreatitis seen through the stomach gas bubble.

B. *Opacities*

Determine the organ of origin.

(1) Kidneys
- cortical - necrosis, chronic glomerulonephritis (both rare causes)
- medullary - papillary necrosis
- localized - opaque stones (calcium or cysteine)
- whole kidney - tuberculous auto-nephrectomy
- stag horn - recurrent infection with urea splitting organism (e.g. proteus)
- tumour mass - either benign or malignant
- diffuse nephrocalcinosis
  - idiopathic hypercalciuria
  - hyperparathyroidism
  - medullary sponge kidney
  - renal tubular acidosis.

(2) Bladder
- stones
- calcium within the wall of the bladder suggests schistosomiasis and despite extensive calcification the bladder is still capable of contraction
- calcium on the surface of a bladder tumour.

(3) Liver
- calcification of old pyogenic or amoebic abscess
- hydatid cysts
- portal venous calcification. The portal vein may calcify after thrombosis, therefore look for an enlarged spleen
- primary and metastatic tumours
- histoplasmosis.

(4) Vascular
- aortic aneurysm. Look at lateral abdominal film and for evidence of generalized atherosclerosis, often most obvious in the pelvic vessels. Ultrasound is a useful confirmatory test.
- splenic venous calcification (typically tortuous in the left upper quadrant), very common in the elderly and of no significance.

(5) Others
- tuberculous mesenteric glands, common

- phleboliths – look like small Polo mints in the pelvic cavity, very common and increase with age
- ovarian cysts. Low X-ray density (that of fat) sometimes containing bone and teeth
- appendicolith – usually in right lower quadrant
- costal cartilages (upper abdomen)
- pancreas – diffuse pancreatic calcification is virtually diagnostic of chronic pancreatitis
- uterine fibroids with blotch (popcorn) calcification
- psoas region associated with spinal deformity suggests tuberculosis
- spleen when calcified suggests tuberculosis
- adrenal, often following haemorrhage and tuberculosis, but the majority of calcified adrenals are idiopathic.

C. *Organs and soft tissues*

(1) Spleen
- when enlarged may displace stomach medially and the splenic colon downwards

(2) Liver
- Reidel's lobe causes enlargement of the right lobe of the liver and is a normal variant
- pulmonary emphysema will cause the liver to be displaced downwards.

(3) Kidneys
- both should be of a length equal to 3.5–4 × the height of an adjacent lumbar vertebral body. They will be within 1.5 cm of each other in length, and their position may vary (i.e. the right kidney not necessarily lower than the left).

(4) Psoas shadows
- may be useful to distinguish retro-peritoneal disease, but in about 15% of normals only one is visible.

(5) Ascites
- usually clinically obvious before detected radiologically. The gut floats medially within the abdomen and the fluid lies peripherally in the loins and in the pelvis. Ultra-sound is better than an abdominal film for the diagnosis.

(6) Pelvic masses
- the full bladder and pregnant or fibroid uterus are the commonest.
(7) Muscle calcification
- parasitic infection
- bismuth, quinine and mercury injections.

D. Bones

Look at *all* the bones.
(1) Spine
- ankylosing spondylitis
- vertebral compression
- rugger jersey - renal osteodystrophy
- metastases destroying pedicles ('one eyed owl').
(2) Pelvis
- Looser's zones
- Paget's disease
- sacro-iliitis
- metastases and myeloma
- hip joints - osteo-arthritis; avascular necrosis (e.g. from analgesic and steroid therapy) and fractures.

Further Reading

Armstrong, P. (1976). Plain abdominal X-ray film in adults. *Br. J. Hosp. Med.*, **15**, 597.

Interpretation of the Skull Radiograph

(1) Most information is available on the lateral film. Therefore, study this first and use the other views to confirm and localize any abnormality.
(2) It is very easy to over-diagnose abnormality of vault bone texture and fractures because there is great variation in the normal texture of the skull vault and the number of suture lines and their positions.
(3) Ensure that skull views are straight before commenting on the position of the pineal.
(4) Now consider:
(a) *Bones of the vault*
(1) Thickening
- normal variation (common)

- hyperostosis frontalis interna - thickening of the internal table, normal in women
- Paget's disease, sclerosis and thickening
- rarer causes
  - dystrophia myotonica
  - acromegaly
  - chronic fluoride poisoning
  - Caffey's disease in babies

(2) Thinning
  - normal variation, particularly in the parietal region where thinning may be extreme
  - underlying brain tumour (rare)
  - chronic sub-dural haematoma (rare)

(3) Holes
  - normal - parietal foramina, venous lakes
  - lytic metastases - breast, bronchus, thyroid, pancreas, bladder
  - myeloma - multiple with no sclerotic margin
  - post surgery - burr holes, flaps and shunts
  - fibrous dysplasia
  - Paget's disease, large lytic areas may be seen early in the disease
  - rarer causes
    - hyperparathyroidism
    - leukaemia, lymphoma
    - eosinophilic granuloma
    - storage disease: Gaucher's, Niemann-Pick
    - haemangioma of the vault
    - hydatid disease
    - encephalocoele
    - leptomeningeal cysts

(4) Sclerosis
  - normal variation
  - metastases: prostate, breast, gut
  - lymphoma
  - Paget's disease
  - fibrous dysplasia
  - solitary osteoma of the vault
  - rare causes
    - haemangioma

- reaction to a meningioma
- primary hyperparathyroidism
- chronic osteomyelitis
- post-radiotherapy necrosis
- tuberous sclerosis

(b) *Sutures*

(1) Increase in width
- raised intracranial pressure in children
- deposition of leukaemic tissue or neuroblastoma

(2) Wormian bones (extra sutures around lambda)
- clydocranial dysostosis
- osteogenesis imperfecta
- cretinism
- hypophosphatasia
- pyknodysostosis
- arrested hydrocephalus

(c) *Pituitary fossa*

(1) Enlargement - usually obvious if gross, but measurements should be taken to calculate the volume of the fossa if there is doubt.

Normal measurements on lateral skull view:

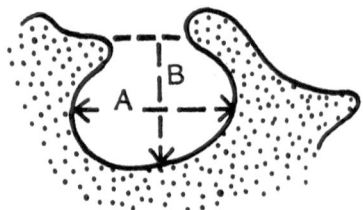

A = AP diameter in mm. (max. 16, min. 5, average 10.6)
B = depth in mm. (max. 12, min. 4, average 8.1)

Comparison of the pituitary fossa seen in a previous film is important as a change is significant. The 'Double Floor' sign may be produced by tipping the head slightly sideways or by asymmetrical pneumatization of the sphenoid sinus and should not be used alone as a sign of fossa enlargement.

(2) Changes of raised intra-cranial pressure -
Thinning of the lamina dura in the pituitary fossa. This is seen at the root of the dorsum sellae initially and then spreads up the dorsum and along the floor (see Figure 3).

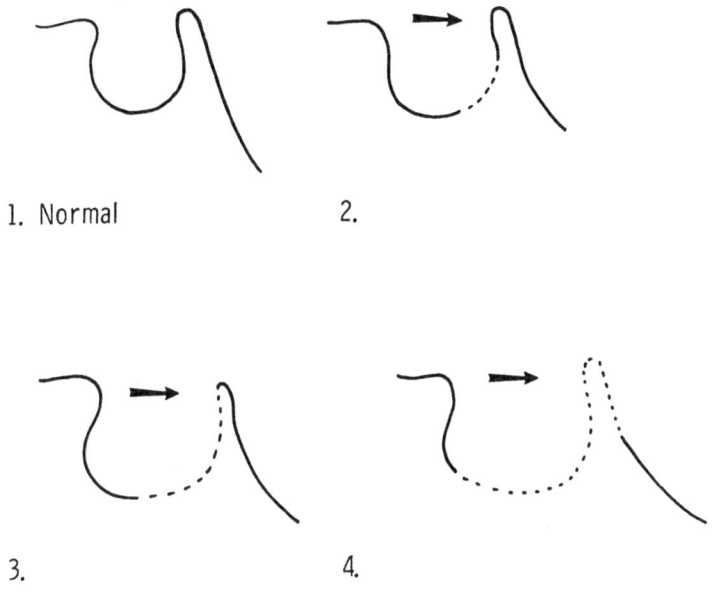

1. Normal   2.

3.   4.

Figure 3 – Changes of pituitary fossa with raised intracranial pressure – progression with time and severity.

(d) *Other changes of raised intra-cranial pressure*

Bone changes will be apparent only after the intra-cranial pressure has been elevated for at least 4 weeks. The early changes are subtle and difficult to distinguish from the changes seen in the elderly.

- thinning of the lesser wings of the sphenoid on AP or PA view of the skull
- widened sutures in children
- increase in interdigitations of the sutures in children
- a shift in the pineal
- a bulging fontanelle can sometimes be seen on the skull film of a baby

Note The copper-beaten appearance of the skull vault is not to be relied upon as a sign of raised intra-cranial pressure, as this may be a variation of normal vault texture

(e) *Enlargement of internal auditory meatus*
- best seen on the Townes or per-orbital view. The maximum diameter of the meatus should not differ by more than 1 mm.

(f) *Intra-cerebral calcification*
(1) Physiological
- pineal
- may be calcified from early adolescence onwards.
- as it lies above the odontoid its midline position is not altered by rotation unless this is excessive. On an AP, PA or Townes view there may be normal variation of 2 mm from the midline position as measured from the *internal* vault surface.
- maximum diameter is 4 mm.
- on the lateral view its normal position is 5 cm perpendicular to a line drawn between the tubercle of the sphenoid and the clivus (see Figure 4).

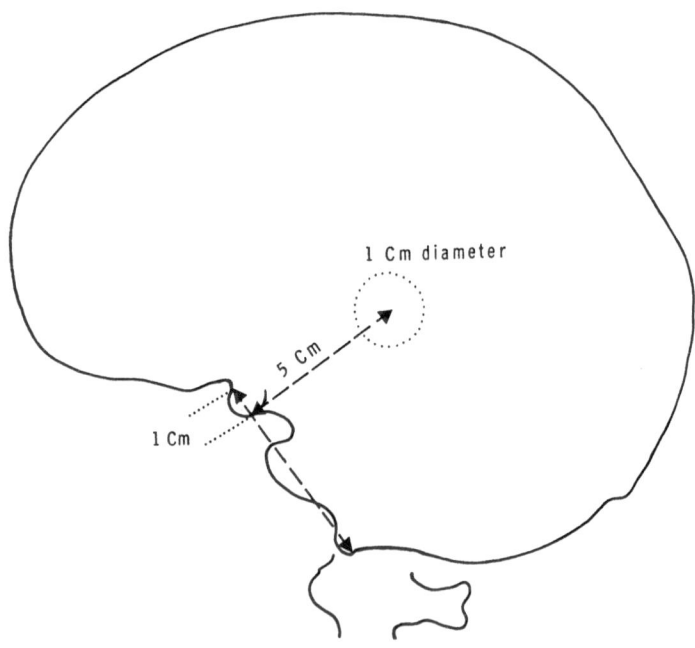

Figure 4 – Position of pineal gland seen on lateral skull view.

- habenular nucleus – 'c'-shaped calcification just in front of the pineal.
- falx and dura, e.g. tentorium.
- choroid plexus – at the confluence of the lateral and posterior horns of the ventricles, usually symmetrical.
- ligaments around the pituitary fossa.

(2) Pathological – see Figure 5.

a) Mid-line and close to mid-line

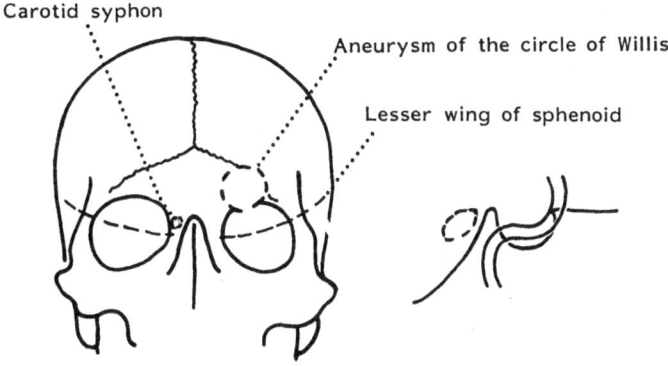

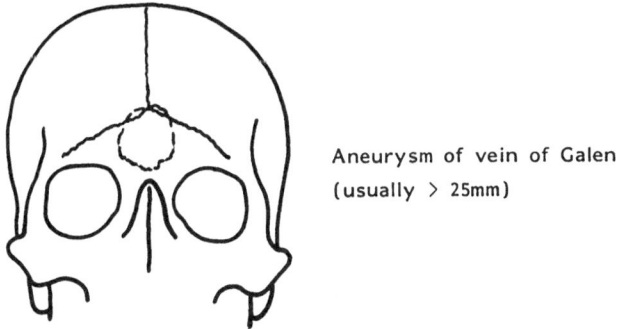

Figure 5 – Pathological calcification on skull radiograph.

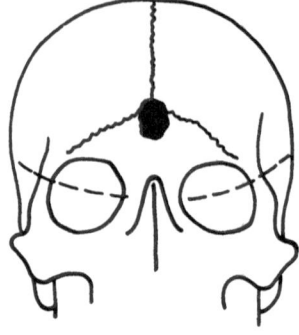

Pineal tumours
(usually >4mm <25mm)

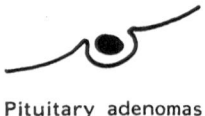

Pituitary adenomas
(1 - 6%)

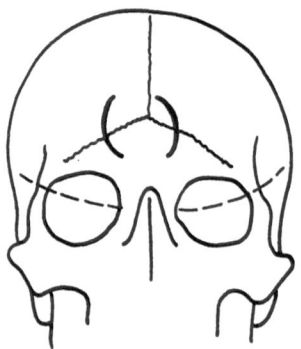

LIPOMA OF CORPUS CALLOSUM

* Classical double "C"

CRANIOPHARYNGIOMAS

* Cystic
* May be large
* Part of rim may calcify
* In or above sella

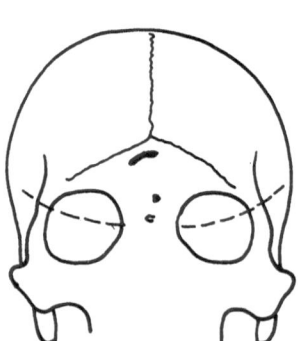

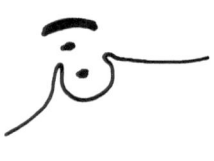

Figure 5,a, continued

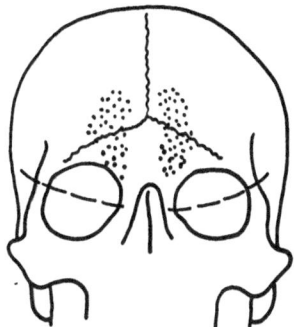

BASAL GANGLIA CALCIFICATION

* Hypoparathyroidism
* Pseudohypoparathyroidism
* Familial

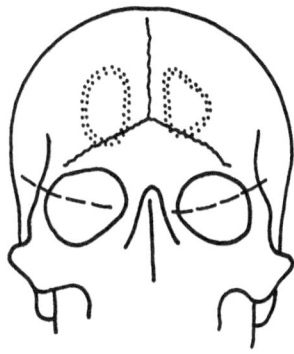

PERIVENTRICULAR

* Toxoplasmosis
* Cytomegalovirus
(with dilated ventricles)

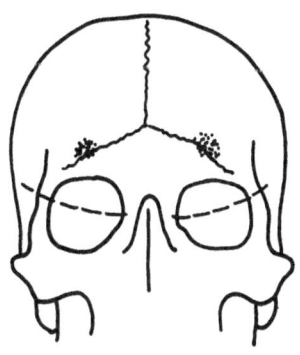

NORMAL CHOROID PLEXUS

Figure 5,a, continued

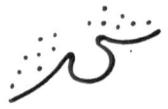

(b) BASE OF SKULL CALCIFICATION

* Tuberculous speckles
* Meningioma
* Aneurysms
* Chordoma

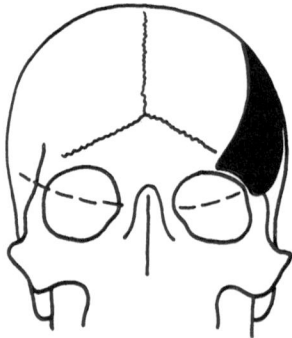

(c) NEAR VAULT

* Meningioma
* Calcified chronic subdural haematoma

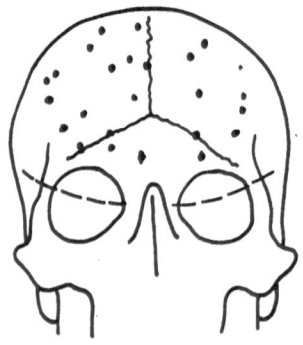

(d) DIFFUSE

* Tuberous sclerosis
* Toxoplasmosis
* Cysticercosis
* Paragonomiasis
* Miliary tuberculosis

Figure 5,b—d

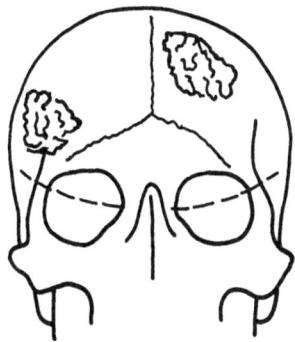

(e) MISCELLANEOUS

* A - V malformations
* Gliomas
* Hamartomas
* Old cerebral abscess

Figure 5,e

(g) *Lumps on the vault*
- sebaceous cyst
- neurofibromatosis
- warts
- encephalocoeles (rare) - look for bone defect
(h) *Soft tissue calcification*
- cysticercosis and other parasites
- calcium at the carotid bifurcation (distinguish from thyroid cartilage)
(i) *Artefacts*
- hair
- curlers
- grips
- plastic beads
- dressings etc.

These may simulate pathological lesions. If in doubt look on more than one film.

Q33

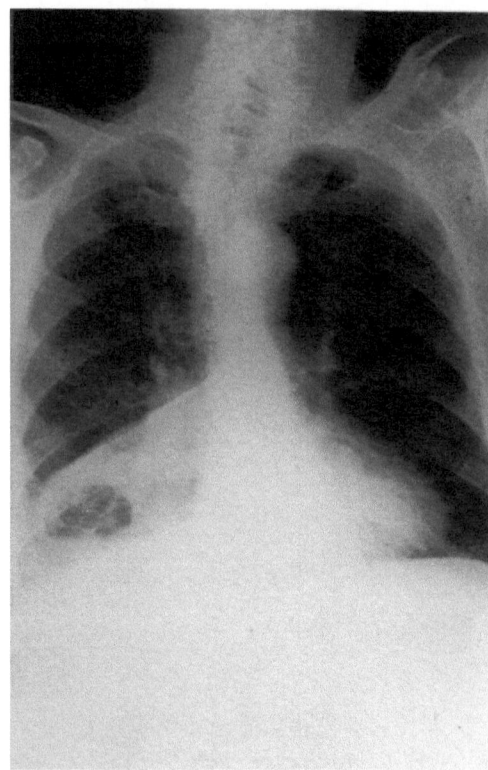

(1) Comment on this chest radiograph.
(2) Suggest a likely diagnosis.

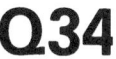

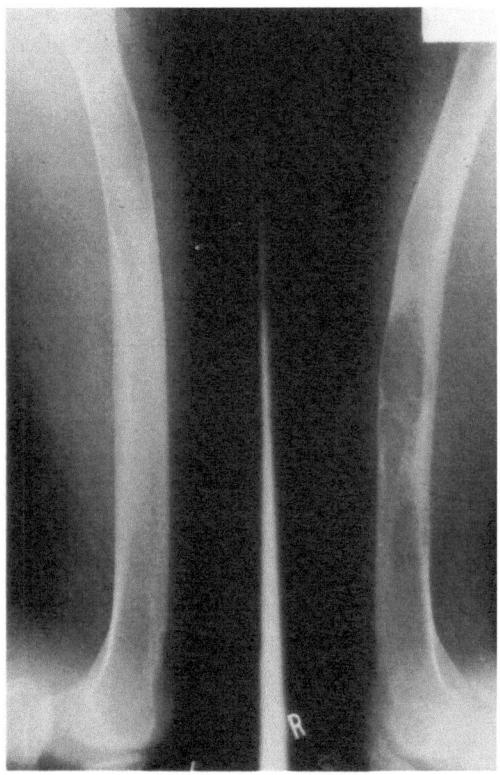

This radiograph shows the femora of a 60-year-old woman who presented with a 4 year history of pain in the legs.

(1) What biochemical investigations would you perform to confirm the diagnosis?
(2) What further radiographs would be helpful for the diagnosis?
(3) What is the likely diagnosis?
(4) What is the radiological differential diagnosis?

Q35

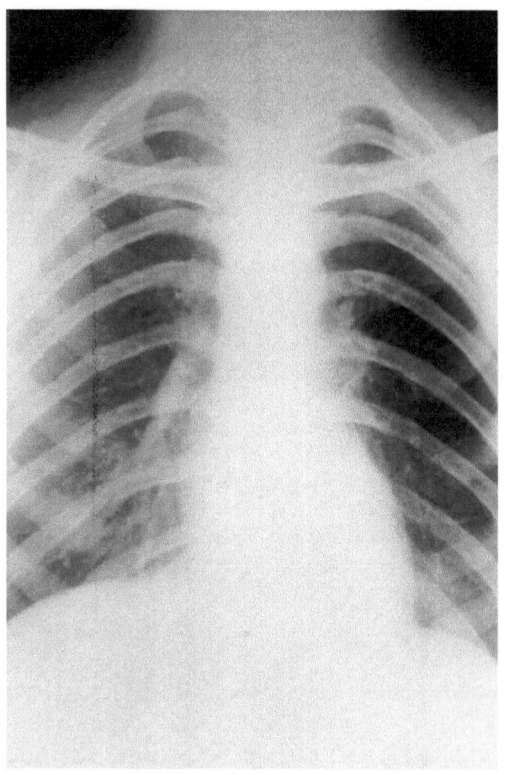

(1) What abnormality is seen in this chest radiograph?
(2) List the possible causes of this appearance.

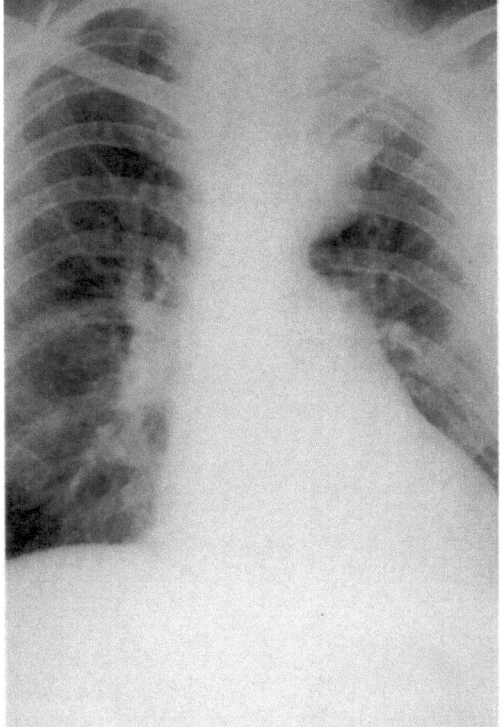

Q36

(1) Give 3 abnormalities seen on this chest radiograph.
(2) Give 3 possible causes of death associated with this condition.

Q37

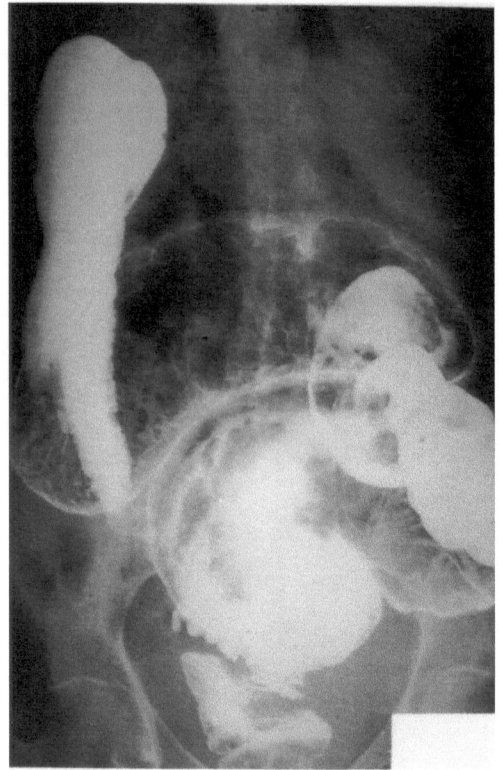

This is a barium enema performed on a 35-year-old man with a pyrexia and a complaint of abdominal pain.

(1) Give 4 radiological abnormalities.
(2) What is the likely diagnosis?

Q38

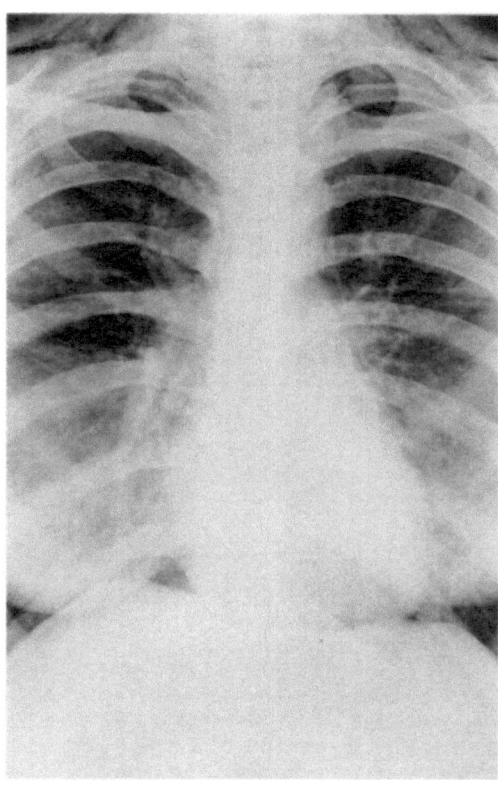

(1) Comment on this chest radiograph which was taken when a 19-year-old labourer with previously diagnosed asthma was admitted with chest pain and shortness of breath.
(2) How would you manage this problem?

Q39

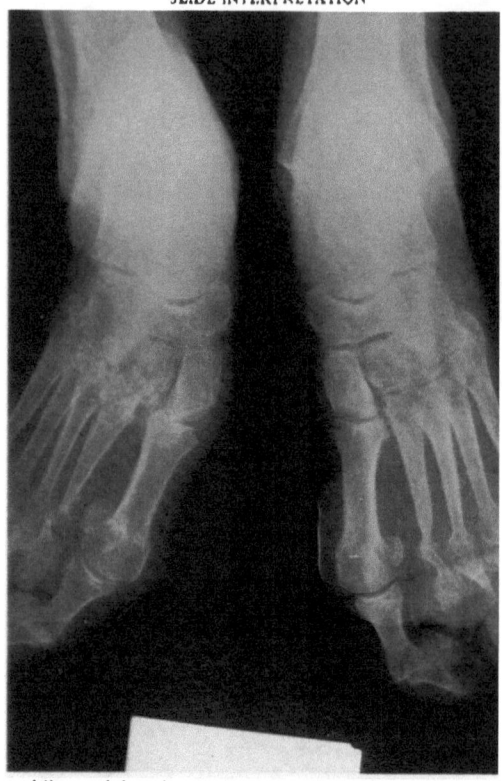

This middle-aged female patient's only specific complaint is of difficulty in walking.

Answers:
(1) What diagnosis is suggested by the radiograph of her feet?
(2) What other abnormal physical signs would you expect in her legs?

Q40

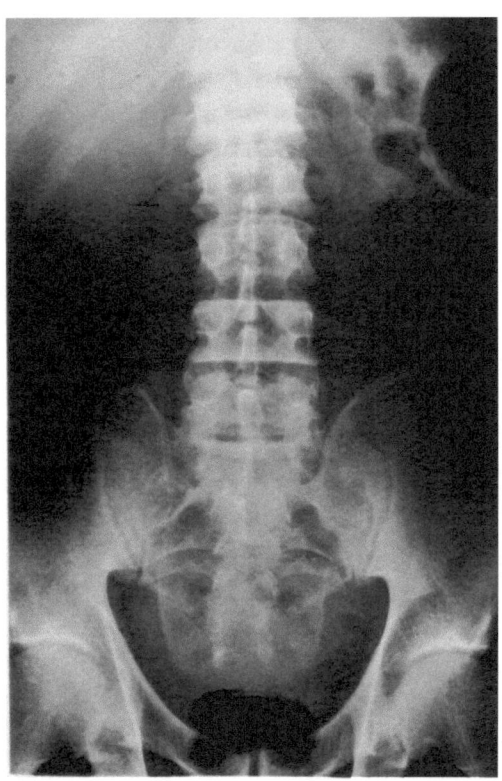

(1) What abnormality is seen on this plain abdominal radiograph?
(2) With what conditions is this abnormality associated?

Q41

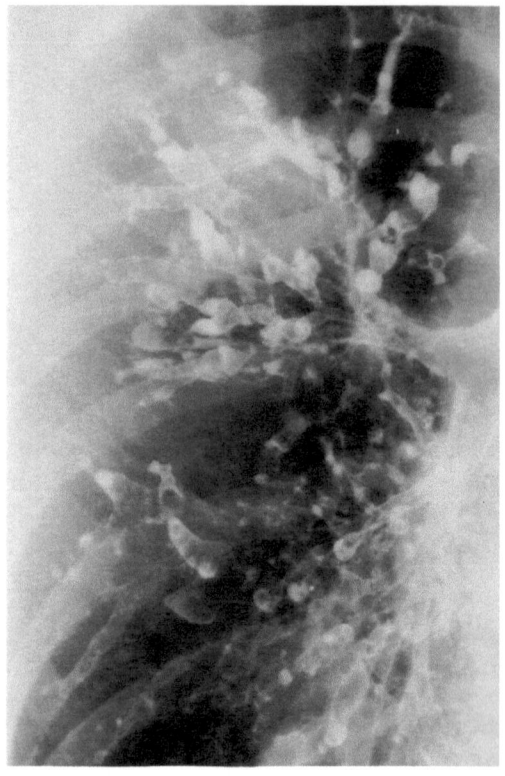

(1) What is the radiological abnormality?
(2) Of which condition is this appearance characteristic?
(3) Give 5 features of this condition.

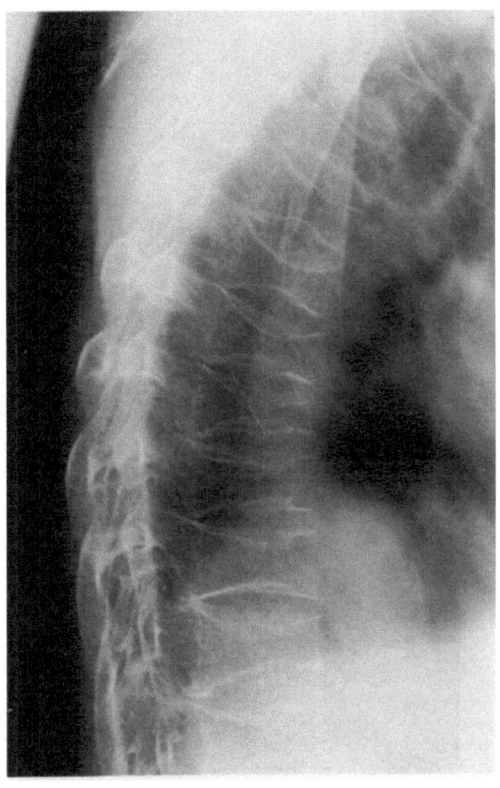

(1) Describe the abnormalities seen in this radiograph.
(2) What is the radiological diagnosis?
(3) What are the causes of this condition?

Q43

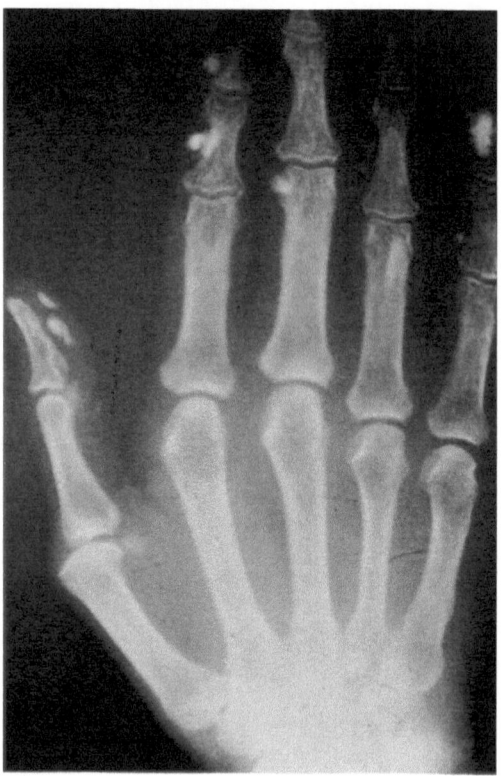

(1) What abnormality do you see on this radiograph?

(2) What is the likely diagnosis?

(3) What abnormalities may be seen on examination of the hand?

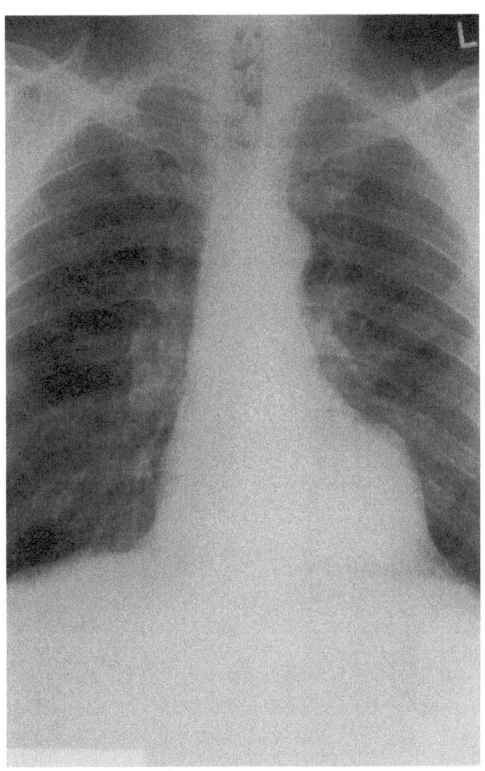

Q44

Three months ago this patient suffered an acute anterior myocardial infarction.

(1) Comment on this chest X-ray suggesting a likely diagnosis.
(2) What abnormalities would you expect to find on his electrocardiogram?
(3) Give 3 indications for surgery.

Q45

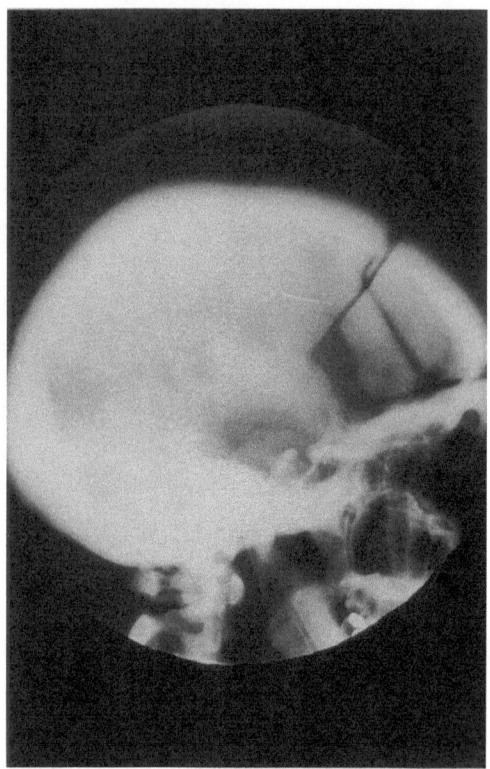

This is a lateral skull X-ray of a 9-year-old girl with anaemia.

(1) What is the diagnosis?
(2) What operation has been performed?
(3) What other complications may be present?

Q46

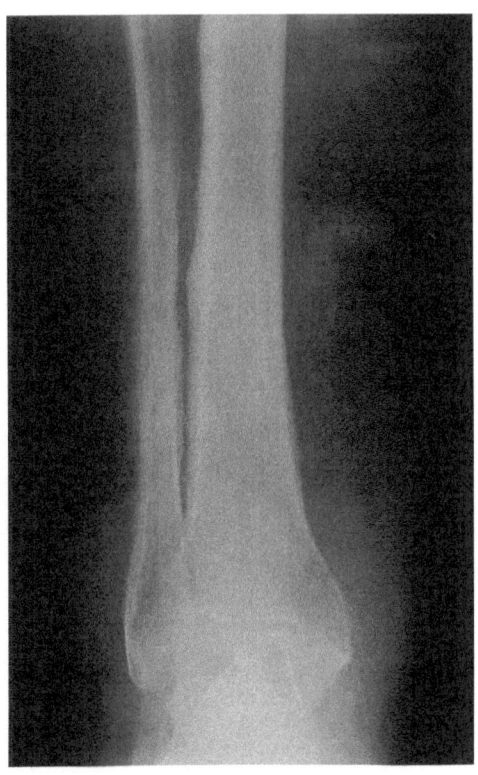

(1) Document two abnormalities seen on this radiograph of the lower leg.
(2) What is the diagnosis?
(3) What is the radiological differential diagnosis of the bony lesion?

Q47

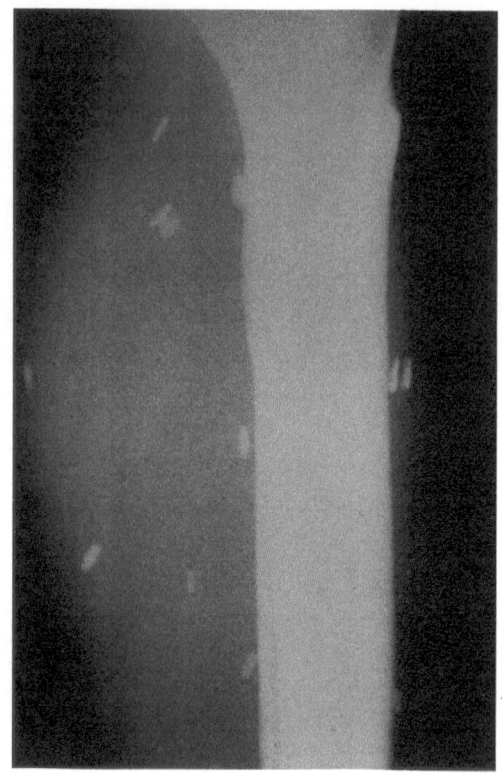

(1) What is the diagnosis?
(2) What is the most likely presentation?
(3) What may a blood film show?
(4) What may stool examination show?

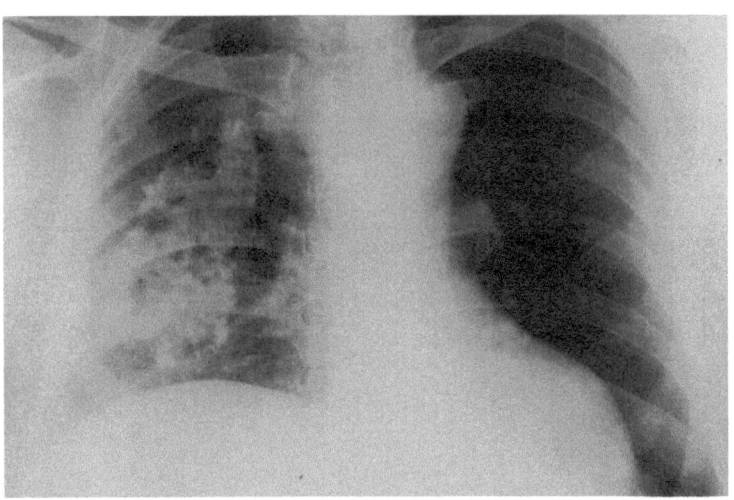

(1) Comment on this chest radiograph.
(2) Give 2 likely diagnoses.

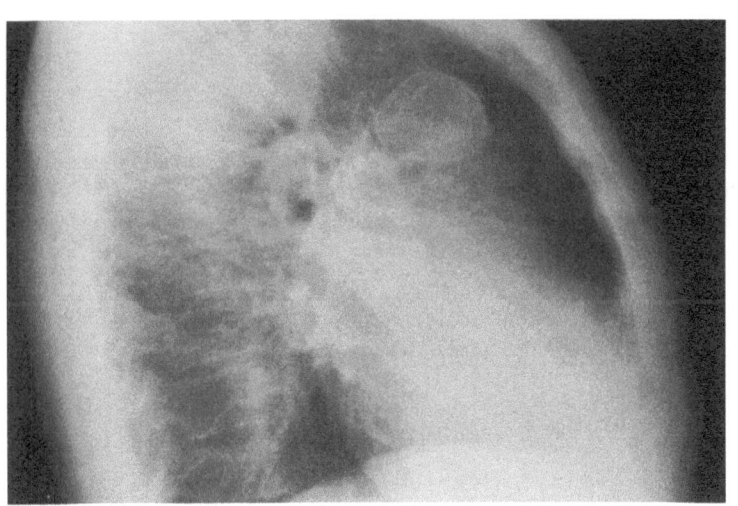

(1) Describe the abnormalities seen on this lateral chest radiograph.
(2) List 4 possible causes.

Q50

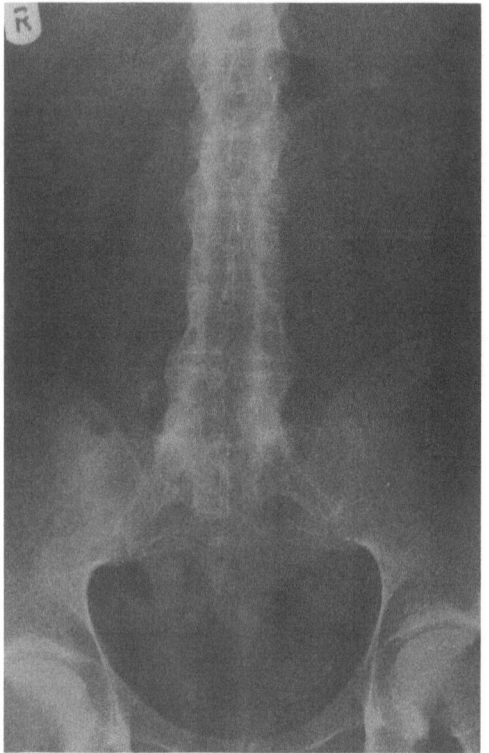

This is an abdominal radiograph of a 60-year-old man with a 30 year history of back pain. He presented with an acute illness consisting of fever, bleeding gums and a severe haemorrhagic sore throat.

(1) Document the abnormal features on the radiograph.
(2) What is the likely cause of his acute illness?

Answers:

A1

(1) This is a jejunal biopsy showing sub-total villous atrophy and crypt hyperplasia. Although the thickness of the mucosa is normal, the ratio of villous height to crypt depth is reversed. Inflammatory cell infiltrate can be seen in the lamina propria. The likely diagnosis is coeliac disease although mild or moderate similar changes may be seen in other diseases of the small bowel.

(2) The biochemical abnormalities will reflect proximal bowel malabsorption. There will be a low serum albumin, calcium, phosphate, folate, iron, magnesium and cholesterol. Plasma potassium is usually low but the total exchangeable body potassium is low. Alkaline phosphatase of bone origin is likely to be elevated in the presence of osteomalacia secondary to malabsorption.

(3) Although the most likely diagnosis from biopsy evidence is coeliac disease the diagnosis can only be firmly established by a trial of a gluten-free diet with assessment of symptoms, normalization of biochemistry, and, if necessary, a further jejunal biopsy which should return towards normal. A subsequent challenge with gluten is usually unnecessary.

Answers:

A2

(1) Short fourth metacarpal.

(2) (a) Pseudo-hypoparathyroidism.
   (b) Pseudo pseudo-hypoparathyroidism.
   (c) Turner's syndrome.
   (d) Noonan's syndrome. There are many similarities with Turner's syndrome (short stature, webbed neck, congenital heart disease), but chromosomes are normal, there is autosomal dominant inheritance and the heart lesion tends to be pulmonary stenosis rather than coarctation of the aorta.

A3

Answers:

(1) Hyperpigmented areas on the gums and buccal mucosa.

(2) Addison's disease.

The precise hormonal basis for the pigmentation is unclear. There is doubt that 'beta MSH' as such is present in the circulation, although it makes up part of the amino acid sequence of larger molecules that are measured as 'immuno-reactive beta MSH'. Empirically the pigmentation is associated with chronic elevation of ACTH and its secretory by-products.

A4

Answers:

(1) (a) Adenoma sebaceum. This appears as orange-red nodules characteristically distributed in the naso-labial folds and occasionally on the cheeks and chin. They are not adenomas of sebaceous glands, but angiofibromas. Adenoma sebaceum is one of the characteristic skin lesions of tuberous sclerosis.

(b) Hirsutism (inappropriate for the boy's age).

(2) Tuberous sclerosis is characterized by the triad of adenoma sebaceum, mental retardation and epilepsy and the hirsutism is secondary to phenytoin therapy.

(3) (a) Shagreen patch. This is a circumscribed area of sub-epidermal fibrosis occurring in the lumbo-sacral area.

(b) Ungual fibromas.

(c) Ovoid patches of hypomelanosis occurring in the skin over the trunk and limbs and looking like the leaf of a Mountain Ash (ash leaf hypomelanosis). These lesions are frequently present at birth, unlike the other skin signs, and may therefore be useful in the differential diagnosis of epilepsy.

(d) Café au lait spots. Similar to those seen in neurofibromatosis.

Answers: **A5**
(1) Lichen planus of the buccal mucosa.

(2) There is a pattern of fine white streaks radiating from a bluish papule a few millimetres in diameter.
Many patients with lichen planus have buccal lesions and these may commonly be the sole manifestation of the disease.

(3) The characteristic skin lesion is a flat, polygonal violaceous papule on the surface of which there may be white dots or lines (Whickham's striae).
Lichen planus may affect any part of the body surface but the commonest areas are:
   (a) flexor aspect of the wrist
   (b) lumbar regions
   (c) ankles
   (d) the palms and soles

Answers: **A6**
Retino-choroiditis involving the macular region due to toxoplasmosis. This is the commonest ocular manifestation of toxoplasmosis and occurs in acute congenital toxoplasmosis but not in acquired infection. The primary focus appears in the retina with secondary reaction in the choroid and occasionally inflammation of the sclera. It is usually bilateral. The acute phase lasts for between 2 and 4 months, followed by atrophy of the choroid and pigment proliferation around the periphery of the lesion. Secondary optic atrophy may occur.

Answers: **A7**
(1) Both specimens of urine have been exposed to ultra-violet light.

(2) Porphyria cutanea tarda. The smaller specimen (belonging to the patient) fluoresces coral pink under ultra-violet light (Wood's light). This fluorescence is due to increased urinary excretion of

uroporphyrins, which when present in very large amounts produce a pink colour even without ultra-violet light. Urinary excretion of porphobilinogen and delta-aminolaevulinic acid is not increased.

(3) These patients have a hereditary partial deficiency of uroporphyrin decarboxylase but clinical manifestations occur only in the presence of acquired liver disease, usually alcoholic cirrhosis or siderosis. Clinical manifestations are limited to the skin and include scarring, hyperpigmentation and hirsutism. Abdominal and neurological manifestations are absent and there is no sensitivity to barbiturates.

(4) Symptoms may be improved by venesection or iron chelation therapy.

A8

Answers:

(1) Erythema nodosum.

(2) (a) In the majority of patients no cause is found (i.e. idiopathic).
    (b) In Britain probably the most common cause is sarcoidosis.
    (c) Streptococcal infection.
    (d) Drugs, particularly sulphonamides (and possibly the contraceptive pill).
    (e) Systemic mycoses (blastomycosis, coccidioidomycosis) particularly seen in the United States.
    (f) Ulcerative colitis, Crohn's disease.
    (g) Viruses (lymphogranuloma venereum, measles and cat scratch fever).
    (h) Malignancy (Hodgkin's and leukaemia) – rare.
    (i) Tuberculosis at the time of development of hypersensitivity (about 6 weeks after inoculation).

Erythema nodosum leprosum should not be included because the distribution and histopathology of the skin lesions are different. Biopsy of the lesions of erythema nodosum shows non-specific vasculitis and the diagnosis must therefore be made clinically.

Answers:

A9

Medullated nerve fibres.

The nerve fibres throughout the retina and in front of the lamina cribosa are usually non-medullated, but occasionally a flare of medullation is seen around the optic disc.

This is a normal variation.

Answers:

A10

(1) Necrobiosis lipoidica diabeticorum.

This is an uncommon but characteristic lesion consisting of a sharply demarcated plaque, an erythematous border and a red-brown centre that becomes yellow as lipids are deposited. Central ulceration with telangiectasia frequently occurs. In over 90% of cases the lesions are pre-tibial but they may also occur on the arms or hands. They occur 3 times more frequently in women than men.

(2) These lesions may antedate the development of clinical diabetes mellitus or occur during the course of the disease. However, there may be no abnormality of glucose tolerance. In patients with established diabetes there is no relationship between the activity of these lesions and blood glucose control.

Answers:

A11

(1) The sclerotics are blue and this is a feature of osteogenesis imperfecta.

(2) Autosomal dominant.

(3) Fractures leading to skeletal deformities, deafness, characteristic triangular facies, aortic root dilatation, mitral valve prolapse.

A12

Answers:

(1) There is distal digital gangrene and fusiform swelling of the fingers.

(2) The rest of the skin of the hands does not look ischaemic which suggests that the gangrene is likely to be due to disease of small vessels. The swelling of the fingers suggests rheumatoid disease as the underlying diagnosis. Arteritis occurs in patients who are sero-positive and who usually also have nodules. The presentation of the arteritis depends on the size of the vessel involved:

    (a) small nail fold lesions.

    (b) skin necrosis – leg ulcers, ulceration over nodules.

    (c) mononeuritis multiplex

    (d) large vessel disease

Other possible causes of this appearance include:

    (a) infective endocarditis

    (b) systemic lupus erythematosus

    (c) recurrent emboli associated with cervical ribs

    (d) mixed cryoglobulinaemia

    (e) hypersensitivity vasculitis

A13

Answers:

(1) The bridge of the nose has collapsed due to destruction of the cartilage. In this case it is most likely to be due to relapsing polychondritis. The chondrocytes degenerate and the cartilage is replaced by fibrous tissue. Cell mediated immunity to cartilage may play a role in the pathogenesis of this disease, but the aetiology is unknown. Disease activity is suppressed by cortico-steroids and recent reports suggest that dapsone may be useful in treatment.

It predominately occurs in middle age with involvement of the ears and nose, in 80–90% of patients.

(2) The disease process may also involve the larynx, trachea, bronchi and aortic valve (leading to aortic regurgitation).

This appearance could also be due to congenital syphilis, trauma, or leprosy.

Answers: **A14**

(1) In the centre of the film is a blast cell. Three nucleated red blood cells are also seen. This is a leuco-erythroblastic picture.

(2) In the presence of disturbed architecture or function of the bone marrow haemopoietic cells fail and anaemia results, often with nucleated red cells and primitive white cells in the peripheral blood. Extra-medullary haemopoiesis occurs in chronic states with massive enlargement of the spleen. The exact mechanism of the suppression of haemopoiesis is not known, as any infiltration of the bone marrow tends to be patchy, often with abundant, apparently normal haemopoietic tissue.

Diagnosis depends on finding abnormalities in bone marrow aspirate or trephine biopsy and sometimes this has to be taken from more than one site.

Causes are

(a) 'Haematological malignancy' – leukaemia, lymphoma, myeloma, myelofibrosis (the presence of teardrop cells in the peripheral blood is suggestive of the latter condition).

(b) Infiltration with metastatic carcinoma.

(c) Osteopetrosis – the leuco-erythroblastic anaemia may not be due to encroachment by bone on the marrow space, but may be a primary disorder of stem cells leading to defective production of osteoblasts and blood precursors.

(d) Lipid storage disease.

(e) Infection – fungal, tuberculous.

(f) Granulomas – sarcoidosis, histiocytosis.

Answers: **A15**

(1) Retinitis pigmentosa.

This is progressive bilateral retinal degeneration for which there is no recognized treatment. The early symptoms are night blindness with constriction of peripheral vision and later deterioration in day vision. The characteristic field defect is an annular scotoma. The disturbance of pigment (often likened to bone corpuscles) is arranged in a circumscribed zone around the fundus and eventually spreads to encroach on the central and peripheral areas. The inheritance of this condition is variable with the dominant form having the best prognosis.

(2) (a) Laurence–Moon–Biedl syndrome (autosomal recessive) – obesity, hypogonadism and mental retardation.
(b) Usher's syndrome (autosomal recessive) – congenital deafness.
(c) Bassen–Kornzweig's syndrome (autosomal recessive) – abetalipoproteinaemia, spinocerebellar degeneration, malabsorption and acanthocytosis.
(d) Refsum's disease (autosomal recessive) – polyneuropathy, ataxia, skeletal deformities, cardiac conduction defects and icthyosis.
(e) Batten's disease (familial amaurotic idiocy) – hereditary neuronal storage disease.

A16 Answers:

(1) There is gross oedema of the whole body (including the face) and a distended abdomen, most likely due to ascites. This appearance is due to hypoproteinaemia, almost certainly from nephrotic syndrome. The typical 'soft' oedema is the result of anti-natiuresis and antidiuresis as an attempt to compensate for hypotonic hypovolaemia. The result is expansion of the extracellular compartment. A pathological diagnosis is made on renal biopsy, although some information may be gained from analysis of urinary proteins and an assessment of the selectivity of protein excretion.

(2) (a) About 80% of children with nephrotic syndrome have 'minimal change lesion' on light microscopy with fusion of podocytes seen on electron microscopy. There is highly selective proteinuria. Hypertension and haematuria may rarely occur, but these findings are usually transient and mild.
(b) Focal glomerulo-sclerosis.
(c) Membrano-proliferative glomerulonephritis.
(d) Other causes of the nephrotic syndrome.

Answers:

A17

(1) There is triangular encroachment of the conjunctiva onto the cornea presenting as a fleshy growth, which when single is usually found on the nasal side and fails to progress beyond the middle of the cornea. The abnormality is a pterygium (Greek for wing). The pterygium may be a primary condition or may be the result of an inflammatory process in which a fold of inflamed conjunctiva is dragged across the cornea behind a progressive ulcer (pseudo-pterygium). In this condition a probe can be passed under the inflammatory lesion, but not under a true pterygium.

(2) There are no symptoms except for slight irritation associated with periods of inflammatory engorgement.

(3) The condition is found in patients exposed to a hot, dry, dusty environment and, therefore, patients tend to be from the Middle East and Australia.

Answers:

A18

(1) Psoriasis. There are small circular pits due to psoriatic foci on the underside of the nail fold which moulds the plate during its formation. Nail growth is increased and onycholysis (separation of the tip of the nail from its bed by a yellowish wad of keratin) is often present.

(2) (a) Characteristic skin lesions.
    (b) Arthropathy. There is a close temporal relationship between psoriatic nail lesions and arthropathy of which 4 types may occur:
       (i) Distal – predominantly terminal inter-phalangeal with associated nail dystrophy (less than 20%)
       (ii) Rheumatoid arthritis type (the commonest form)
       (iii) Sacro-iliac joint involvement with spondylitis (20%)
       (iv) Arthritis mutilans (5%)

A19

Answers:

(1) Acanthosis nigricans. There is hyperpigmentation (often in areas of multiple confluent papillomas) resulting in a velvety elevation of the surface of the epidermis. Pruritus may be a feature. The lesions typically involve the axilla, groin, umbilicus and nipples but more extensive lesions may occur.

(2) (a) Internal malignancy – usually adenocarcinoma (60% gastric). Occasionally squamous cell carcinoma or lymphoma.
(b) Endocrine disorders – insulin-resistant diabetes mellitus, Cushing's syndrome, acromegaly, polycystic ovary syndrome.
(c) Congenital.
(d) Partial lipodystrophy.

A20

Answers:

(1) Generalized gingival hyperplasia.

(2) (a) Long-term phenytoin therapy. This may affect up to 40% of patients on long-term treatment and poor oral hygiene may contribute to the hyperplasia. Other anti-convulsant drugs are generally free of this effect. Folate supplementation may help the hyperplasia.
(b) Myelomonocytic leukaemia.
(e) Gingival hyperplasia may be a familial condition.
(d) Cyclosporin therapy has been implicated and there are case reports of the association of gingival hyperplasia with several conditions (Wegener's granulomatosis, tuberous sclerosis untreated with anticonvulsant therapy).

Localized gingival hyperplasia (epulis) may be due to recurrent inflammation or trauma.

Answers:

A21

(1) Many of the red blood cells appear large and in these cells there is a central pink nodule separated from an outer pink ring by a circular area of pallor - target cells. These cells are characterized by visual macrocytosis, but the measured mean corpuscular volume is normal; a surface area to volume ratio greater than normal, either due to a reduction in the contents of the cell or an increase in surface area; and increased resistance to lysis by hypotonic solutions.

(2) Target cells will be formed in conditions leading to a reduction in red cell volume or to an increase in surface membrane.
   (a) Hyposplenism - young red blood cells have a high membrane to cytoplasm ratio, and in the spleen they lose membrane as they become mature.
   (b) Deficient production of haemoglobin - thalassaemia, HbC disease and HbC trait.
   (c) Liver disease, particularly associated with cholestasis. Red cell membrane lipids are in equilibrium with plasma lipids and when there is a disturbance of plasma lipids (associated with cholestasis) there may be an increase in red cell membrane lipids and an increase in membrane surface area.
   (d) Conditions associated with abnormal lecithin cholesterol acyl transferase (LCAT). A deficiency of this enzyme allows accumulation of lipid in the membrane.

Answers:

A22

(1) Left parotid enlargement.

(2) (a) Mumps. This is probably the commonest cause of unilateral parotid enlargement. This almost invariably progresses to bilateral involvement, but one side may precede the other by 4–6 days.
   (b) Sarcoidosis.
   (c) Mikulicz's syndrome, Sjögren's syndrome.
   (d) Chronic alcoholism.
   (e) Bacterial parotitis. This may be associated with a stone in Stenson's duct, or occur post-operatively associated with

dehydration. There would be severe pain and the skin over-lying the gland would be hyperaemic.

(f) Parotid gland tumour – involvement of the facial nerve with lower motor neurone paralysis would make this diagnosis more likely.

(g) Lymphoma involving the parotid gland.

A23

Answers:

(1) Onycholysis (separation of the nail from its bed). The brown-black discoloration of the nails may be due to accumulation of dirt under the nail plate, but may also be due to secondary bacterial infection with *Pseudomonas* which produces a green–black discolouration.

(2) (a) Trauma, usually repeated minor trauma, often associated with occupation. Repeated maceration with water is also a cause. 'Idiopathic' onycholysis may be due to unrecognized trauma.

(b) Psoriasis.

(c) Fungal infections.

(d) 'Bacterial infections' particularly with *Pseudomonas*, although this is a complication of nail plate separation rather than a cause.

(e) Impaired peripheral circulation.

(f) Yellow-nail-syndrome. The nail is yellow and separated from its bed due to oedema caused by an abnormality of the lymphatics. This abnormality may also lead to bilateral pleural effusions. ,

(g) Hyperthyroidism (Plummer's nails).

(h) Drugs. Onycholysis has been described with cloxacillin and cephaloridine therapy (in patients with renal failure) and with demeclocycline. This may be a photosensitivity reaction as onycholysis has also been reported following treatment with benoxaprofen.

Answers:

A24

(1) There is pallor of the optic disc suggesting optic atrophy, but in addition there is pallor of the whole fundus and the retinal arteries are narrow and thread-like. The retinal veins are also narrower than normal. These appearances are due to central retinal artery occlusion.

The macula is often easily seen because ganglion cells are lacking in this area and the choroid is visible through the thin fovea. Also the cilio-retinal artery which supplies the macula may be preserved when the central retinal arteries are occluded.

(2) (a) Retinal artery embolism from the heart or major vessels.
   (b) Arteritis, e.g. giant cell arteritis, Behçet's disease.
   (c) Contributory factors include increased blood viscosity, glaucoma, reduced pressure in the retinal blood vessels and 'spasm' of the retinal artery.

Answers:

A25

(1) Achondroplasia.

(2) (a) Short stature with normal sexual development – excludes pituitary dwarfism.
   (b) The short stature is due to short limbs with relatively normal development of the spine. Sitting height tends to be normal and measurement of crown to pubis height is greater than pubis to heel. The shortness of the limbs is more noticeable proximally (humerus and femur).
   (c) Apparently large forehead.
   (d) Normal intelligence.
   (e) Normal plasma chemistry with the patient taking no treatment excludes rickets.
   (f) No evidence of fracture excludes osteogenesis imperfecta as a cause for short limbs.

A26 Answers:
(1) (a) 'Half and half nails'. The proximal nailbed is white and the distal nailbed brown. This abnormality was described by Lindsay in association with chronic renal failure and is also known as 'renal nails'.
(b) Clubbing of the fingers. In the context of chronic renal failure this should be called 'pseudo-clubbing' and is due to expansion of the terminal phalanges by the bone changes of hyperparathyroidism.

(2) Chronic renal failure.

A27 Answers:
(1) There is loss of subcutaneous fat in a clearly demarcated symmetrical distribution in the lower part of the body, stopping at mid-thigh. This is characteristic of partial lipodystrophy. In this condition there is a dystrophic process involving loss of subcutaneous fat which usually starts at the face and works downwards symmetrically, but may start at the feet and work upwards. 80% of patients are female and in most cases the loss of subcutaneous fat starts at the age of about 15 years. The skin is normal, but the veins and muscles appear hypertrophied because of the loss of fat.

A diagnosis which might be considered is bilateral rupture of quadriceps tendons, but it is possible to see the patella in the normal position and wrinkles of skin above the patella suggesting normal muscle tone.

Insulin therapy, causing either lipo-atrophy (lower thigh) or lipohypertrophy (upper thigh) is most unlikely as a cause of this appearance.

(2) (a) Hypertriglyceridaemia.
(b) Insulin resistance leading to overt diabetes mellitus in 20% of cases.
(c) Glomerulonephritis with reduced complement levels. There is activation of complement by the alternative pathway in association with C3 nephritic factor.
(d) Acanthosis nigricans.

Answers:

A28

(1) Optic atrophy. There is marked pallor of the disc, with no abnormality of the vessels and retina. The red colour of the normal disc is related to the number and fullness of the capillaries in the nerve head. Anaemia and ischaemia may result in pallor of the optic disc. The diagnosis of optic atrophy depends more on loss of visual acuity and field than the disc colour. Destruction of the nerve fibres and subsequent gliosis is the principal cause of the pallor of the atrophic disc. In the primary form there is a uniform shallow cupping of the disc as a result of the disappearance of nerve fibres and longitudinal shrinkage. If the atrophy is preceded by papillitis or papilloedema (secondary) the normal cupping of the disc may be filled by proliferative glial tissue.

(2) Optic atrophy is associated with the following conditions:
- (a) Injury or ischaemia of the optic nerve (including pressure from tumours of nerve, bone or pituitary gland).
- (b) Neurosyphilis. This is the cause in 20% of patients with tabes dorsalis.
- (c) Exogenous toxins, such as chemicals and tobacco.
- (d) Following acute retrobulbar neuritis (this frequently affects only the temporal half).
- (e) Following papilloedema.
- (f) Secondary to inflammatory or degenerative retinal disease.
- (g) Hereditary (Leber's disease).
- (h) Severe blood loss may occasionally be followed by optic atrophy.

Answers:

A29

(1) Rheumatoid nodules.

These are non-tender and usually found over pressure points such as the extensor surface of the ulna at the elbow, the Achilles tendon or the ischial tuberosities. Usually subcutaneous, they may also be intracutaneous, adherent to the periosteum or may form within tendons. Small vessel vasculitis is thought to be the initiating event in their formation. Similar nodules may be found in the heart, pericardium or lungs.

The differential diagnosis includes tuberous xanthomata, tophaceous gout, the nodules seen in rheumatic fever and possibly those seen in systemic lupus erythematosus.

The joint changes of rheumatoid arthritis may be seen in this patient's hand.

(2) Rheumatoid nodules are found in about 20% of patients with rheumatoid arthritis at some time during the course of their disease. They are found only in patients with a positive test for rheumatoid factor and they may disappear during remission. Patients with rheumatoid arthritis fall into 2 main groups. One group has predominantly synovial involvement and a good general prognosis, but may develop deforming arthritis. The other group has rheumatoid nodules and may have vasculitis and features of other auto-immune disease. These findings are associated with a poorer prognosis.

A30

Answers:

(1) Malarial ring forms (the early trophozoite stage of plasmodium).

(2) Accurate determination of the species of plasmodium is often difficult from a peripheral blood film. Female crescent-shaped gametocytes occurring free from the red cells are diagnostic of falciparum. Stages later than the early trophozoite stage are not seen in falciparum infestation as these tend to be sequestered in the capillaries and do not appear in the peripheral blood. The ring forms of falciparum appear as small (smaller than the 3 other species) blue rings with single or double red chromatin dots. Falciparum parasitizes red cells of all ages and, therefore, the infestation is heavy with red cells occasionally containing 2 parasites. Heavy parasitaemia with one red cell containing 2 parasites is seen on this blood film and suggests infestation with *Plasmodium falciparum*.

A31

Answers:

(1) Administration of tetracycline at the time of odontogenesis. Tetracycline binds avidly to forming bones and teeth and leads to diffuse yellow-brown staining of the teeth which fluoresce in ultra-violet light.

(2) (a) Haemolytic disease at the time of odontogenesis (for example sickle cell disease, thalassaemias and haemolytic disease of the new born).
   (b) Dentinogenesis imperfecta – leads to discoloration of the teeth, but this is usually associated with dysmorphogenesis.
   (c) Fluorosis – this usually leads to more patchy discoloration.
   (d) A group of hereditary enamel hypoplasias.

A32

Answers:

(1) Vitiligo. The slide shows sharply defined patches of depigmentation which are due to destruction of melanocytes.

(2) (a) Type II (non-insulin dependent) diabetes mellitus.
   (b) Auto-immune thyroid disease.
   (c) Pernicious anaemia.
   (d) Gastric carcinoma.
   (e) Auto-immune hypo-adrenalism.
   (f) Alopecia areata.
Note that thyroid antibodies are present in 20% and parietal cell antibodies in 10% of patients with vitiligo.

A33

Answers:

(1) The radiograph shows an abscess cavity in the right lower zone. There is also consolidation and loss of volume of the right lower lobe. The right hilum is probably enlarged.

(2) The association of loss of lung volume with consolidation and abscess formation suggests the presence of a proximal obstruction, probably due to a bronchial neoplasm.

A34 Answers:

(1) (a) Plasma calcium, phosphate, chloride, bicarbonate and immu-noreactive parathyroid hormone. These values may help to make a diagnosis of hyperparathyroidism.

(b) Steroid suppression test may be useful but some patients with hyperparathyroidism and bone disease show suppression of calcium after treatment with hydrocortisone.

(2) (a) Hands may show subperiosteal erosions and 'tufting' of the terminal phalanges.

(b) Skull X-ray may have the 'pepper pot' appearance and show evidence of absorption of the lamina dura.

(3) Osteitis fibrosa cystica (hyperparathyroidism).

(4) (a) Fibrous dysplasia
(b) Myeloma
(c) Eosinophilic granuloma (wrong age group)
(d) Metastases (unlikely but should not be excluded)
(e) Paget's disease of bone in lytic phase
(f) Simple bone cyst (usually solitary).

A35 Answers:

(1) There is increased transradiancy of the left hemithorax.

(2) Having excluded pneumothorax and rotation of the patient, the the following may cause this appearance:

(a) Compensatory emphysema or large emphysematous bulla.

(b) Hyperinflation due to proximal obstruction with peripheral air trapping in expiration.

(c) Massive pulmonary embolus.

(d) Macleod's syndrome. This is congenital or acquired damage to the growing lung leading to hypoplasia particularly of the blood vessels.

(e) Abnormality of the chest wall – mastectomy, congenital absence of pectoralis major (the diagnosis in this case) and polio (wasting of an upper limb may be seen).

Answers:

A36

(1) (a) Cardiomegaly.
   (b) Double aortic knuckle.
   (c) Bilateral notching of the inferior surfaces of ribs (Dock's sign). This may be seen in neurofibromatosis and chronic obstruction of the superior vena cava, but when seen in combination with the other abnormalities it is diagnostic of coarctation of the aorta.

(2) (a) Heart failure due to hypertension.
   (b) Infective endocarditis (either on an associated bicuspid aortic valve or on an area of aortitis below the coarctation).
   (c) Rupture of the aorta.
   (d) Cerebral haemorrhage due to:
      (i) mycotic aneurysm from infective endocarditis.
      (ii) berry aneurysm (associated with coarctation).
      (iii) hypertension.

Answers:

A37

(1) (a) Mucosal ulceration of the descending colon.
   (b) Abnormal dilatation of the transverse colon.
   (c) Pseudo-polyps of the transverse colon.
   (d) Free gas in the peritoneal cavity (above the transverse colon and under the liver).

The ascending colon and caecum are normal in diameter and contain faeces, and are thus unlikely to be involved in the colitic process.

(2) Toxic dilatation of the colon with perforation, probably due to inflammatory bowel disease.

   The transverse colon is abnormally dilated, but the diagnosis of 'toxic dilatation' is a clinical one. The combination of this radiological appearance with fever and abdominal pain strongly suggests this diagnosis.

   The mucosal ulceration in the descending colon with pseudo-polyps, dilatation of the transverse colon and the relative normality of the ascending colon and caecum suggest ulcerative colitis as the diagnosis.

A38 Answers:
(1) The chest X-ray shows mediastinal and subcutaneous emphysema. The muscle planes in the neck can be seen clearly as they are dissected by air. There is no evidence of pneumothorax.

The most likely cause in a patient with asthma is pneumo-mediastinum which is thought to be caused by rupture of the alveolar basement membrane in association with increased intra-alveolar pressure. There is leakage of air into the peri-vascular sheaths and thence into the mediastinum. Spontaneous rupture of the oesophagus is a differential diagnosis. Pneumomediastinum is seen in conditions in which intra-thoracic pressure is increased, such as asthma and labour.

(2) Treatment is directed towards reduction of the intra-alveolar pressure by reducing air-flow obstruction and avoiding intermittent positive pressure ventilation. Treatment other than this conservative approach is rarely required, but in one reported case incision of the muscles of the neck (in order to perform a tracheostomy) led to release of the trapped subcutaneous air and an improvement in the patient's condition.

A39 Answers:
(1) There is disorganization of the bones of the fore-foot. There is splintering and fragmentation of bones of the distal metatarsals and proximal phalanges characterized by distal tapering of bone and osteopenia.

These radiological features are characteristic of diabetic fore-foot osteolysis. This is seen in patients with long-standing diabetes and is usually associated with chronic sensory peripheral neuropathy. There may be evidence of vascular calcification in the foot which makes the diagnosis of diabetes almost certain. This radiological appearance may be seen in certain other forms of chronic sensory peripheral neuropathy, particularly leprosy.

The lower leg is affected in 3 ways in diabetes:
(a) Large joints (Charcot) particularly ankle, tarsal and metatarsal joints and only rarely the hip or knee (unlike syphilis). The joints are hyper-mobile with synovial thickening.

144

(b) Fore-foot osteolysis, where there is progressive destruction of the bones of the fore-foot but prognosis for painless function of the foot is good.

(c) Perforating ulcers of the plantar surface of the fore-foot with associated sepsis. It is important to identify interstitial gas associated with sepsis and osteomyelitis.

(2) There will be signs of diabetic peripheral neuropathy and the foot is likely to be swollen. There may be signs suggestive of acute inflammation and painless hyper-mobility of the fore-foot.

N.B., a neuropathic knee joint suggests tabes dorsalis and shoulder joint syringomyelia.

A40

Answers:

(1) There are discrete triangular areas of calcification overlying the right kidney which are distributed in a semi-circle around the cortico-medullary junction. Close inspection shows that at least one of these opacities has a lucent centre. This appearance is characteristic of renal papillary necrosis.

(2) A reduction in blood supply to the normally very vascular renal papilla leads to its necrosis and calcification. Subsequently there may be cortical atrophy leading to renal failure. Conditions associated with renal papillary necrosis are:

(a) analgesic nephropathy.

(b) diabetes mellitus.

(c) sickle cell disease and trait (and possibly other haemoglobinopathies).

(d) acute ureteric obstruction.

(e) acute pyelonephritis. (It may be that (d) and (e) must occur together before renal papillary necrosis occurs.)

(f) severe hypotension particularly in babies (associated with dehydration or sepsis).

(g) industrial exposure to ethyleneimine.

(h) polyarteritis nodosa.

Renal tuberculosis in the early stages may produce localized lesions which are initially radiologically indistinct from renal papillary necrosis, but which do not become diffuse and bilateral.

A41 **Answers:**
(1) Proximal saccular bronchiectasis.

(2) Allergic broncho-pulmonary aspergillosis.
Aspergillosis may produce disease of 4 types:
(a) colonization of previously damaged lung-tissue – aspergilloma
(b) allergic broncho-pulmonary aspergillosis
(c) invasion of tissues, particularly in immuno-compromised hosts
(d) intoxication with aflatoxin.

(3) This condition may be present in up to 20% of patients with asthma. It is caused by hypersensitivity to aspergillus species (usually *A. fumigatus*).
The following are features:
(a) positive aspergillus skin test.
(b) increase in serum IgE (both specific and non-specific).
(c) precipitating antibodies demonstrable in the serum.
(d) episodic bronchospasm.
(e) peripheral blood eosinophilia.
(f) radiological evidence of transient or fixed pulmonary infiltrates.
(g) proximal saccular bronchiectasis.

A42 **Answers:**
(1) (a) Decreased bone density. This is a poor sign of osteopenia as up to 50% of bone mineral may be lost before there is any noticeable rarefaction. Bone density is also very difficult to assess.
(b) Cortical thinning with the cortex of normal density but appearing sclerotic when compared with the rest of the bone.
(c) Biconcave compression of the vertebral end plates which are intact.
(d) Compression fractures of the vertebral bodies with the apex of the wedge anteriorly. A vertebral wedge fracture with the apex posteriorly suggests malignancy.
(e) Prominence of vertical and loss of horizontal trabeculae.

(2) Osteoporosis.

(3) (a) idiopathic (senile, postmenopausal or juvenile)
    (b) sex hormone deficiency
    (c) thyrotoxicosis
    (d) hypercorticolism (including iatrogenic)
    (e) myeloma
    (f) leukaemia
    (g) hyperparathyroidism
    (h) disuse
    (i) long-term heparin therapy
    (j) connective tissue disorders (Marfan's, Ehlers–Danlos) and homocystinuria
    (k) chronic liver disease.

Answers:

A43

(1) Calcification of the subcutaneous tissue of the fingers, particularly distally.

(2) Scleroderma. A group of patients with scleroderma is recognized in whom systemic involvement is minimal but cutaneous involvement is prominent. These patients manifest calcinosis, Raynaud's phenomenon, oesophageal motility disturbances, sclerodactyly and telangiectasia – CREST syndrome. When the digital calcification is widespread, the eponym Thibierge–Weissenbach syndrome may be used.

(3) Inspection of the hands may reveal
    (a) evidence of Raynaud's phenomenon.
    (b) thickening and tightening of the skin leading to decreased mobility of the fingers.
    (c) dermal atrophy with shiny skin.
    (d) ulceration leading to gangrene and eventually auto-amputation of digits.
    (e) pulp atrophy and resorption of the fingertips.
    (f) subcutaneous calcification.
    (g) depigmentation or hyperpigmentation.
    (h) hair loss.

A44 Answers:

(1) The left heart border is abnormal in contour and suggests left ventricular aneurysm.

(2) There may be changes of transmural, anterior myocardial infarction (Q waves and inverted T waves in the antero-lateral chest leads) and in addition persistent elevation of ST segments in these leads.

(3) Aneurysmectomy may be considered if there is:
   (a) cardiac failure resistant to medical treatment.
   (b) recurrent dysrhythmias resistant to medical treatment.
   (c) recurrent systemic embolization.

A45 Answers:

(1) The bone appears very dense with obliteration of the medullary cavity by cortex. This appearance is characteristic of osteopetrosis (marble bone disease) which was described by Albers-Schönberg in 1904. The differential diagnosis of the radiological appearance would include sclerotic metastases and fluorosis.

(2) Osteopetrosis probably results from a primary developmental abnormality of the primordial cell which differentiates to form cellular elements of bone and blood. Defective osteoclastic bone resorption leads to the radiological appearances and to encroachment of bone upon cranial foramina with associated cranial nerve damage. This girl had progressive visual failure with optic atrophy and a frontal craniotomy was performed to decompress the optic nerves.

(3) (a) Recurrent infection, particularly of the mandible following dental treatment, probably caused by defective circulating phagocyte function.
   (b) Cranial nerve damage leading to deafness and blindness; nasal obstruction.
   (c) Defective stem cells may cause bone marrow failure with anaemia, thrombocytopenia and evidence of extra-medullary haemopoiesis (hepato-splenomegaly). It is unlikely that this bone marrow failure is caused solely by encroachment of bone into the marrow space.

(d) Recurrent fractures. The bone is brittle and chalky (rather than being hard and like marble) but the fractures heal well.

(e) Growth failure.

The condition is inherited as an autosomal recessive (malignant juvenile form with death within the first decade as a result of complications of bone marrow failure) or a more benign, autosomal dominant adult form associated with a normal lifespan and no haematological abnormalities.

Answers:

A46

(1) (a) Periosteal new bone formation of the lateral side of the fibula.

(b) Extensive loss of soft tissue overlying the abnormal periosteum.

(2) Varicose ulceration of the leg.

(3) Periosteal new bone formation may be generalized or localized.

(a) Generalized.
  (i) Sickle cell disease.
  (ii) Leukaemia particularly in children.
  (iii) Rheumatoid arthritis, polyarteritis nodosa (particularly seen in bones underlying skin lesions or adjacent to affected joints).
  (v) Syphilis, both congenital and acquired.

(b) Localized.
  (i) Hypertrophic pulmonary osteoarthropathy.
  (ii) Subperiosteal haemorrhage associated with healing fracture and stress fracture (an important differential from primary tumour) and associated with trauma. When seen in several areas in children suggests 'battered baby syndrome'.
  (iii) Bone tumours, both primary and (more rarely) secondary.
  (iv) Osteomyelitis.
  (v) Varicose veins and venous ulceration (a combination of hypoxia and infection).
  (vi) Caffey's syndrome. This is seen in young babies and may be confused with battering.

A47

Answers:

(1) Cysticercosis. The ova of *Taenea solium* (pork tapeworm) when ingested by man result on their death in the formation of calcified cysts in the subcutaneous tissue, brain, muscle, eye, heart, liver and lung (in that order of frequency). The cysts are a few millimetres in length, elliptical in shape and lie with their long axes in the planes of the muscle fibres. The beef tapeworm (*Taenea saginata*) almost never causes cysticercosis.

(2) Epilepsy. The invasive phase is associated with fever and eosinophilia and other symptoms develop many years after this. These symptoms are usually related to cerebral involvement – cysts in other sites are usually asymptomatic.

(3) Eosinophilia.

(4) Taenia eggs and segments. Cysticercosis is usually caused by external auto-infection with the adult worm causing no symptoms in the small intestine. The worm may still (rarely) be *in situ* at the time of presentation of cysticercosis.

A48

Answers:

(1) (a) There is an old fracture of the left clavicle.
   (b) There is diffuse calcification in the right hemithorax.
   (c) Pleural thickening is noted laterally on the right.
   (d) There is elevation of the right hemidiaphragm.

(2) The calcification (almost certainly pleural) and elevated right hemidiaphragm suggest tuberculosis as the most likely cause. This appearance may be seen following haemothorax, and the old fracture of the left clavicle suggests the possibility of trauma to account for this (although old fractures of the clavicle are a common radiological finding).
   Other causes of pleural calcification are unlikely.

Answers:

(1) The radiograph shows a calcified mass in the superior medias-tinum, situated anteriorly.

A49

(2) (a) thymic tumour – if calcification occurs it does so as a peripheral ring as seen in this radiograph

(b) retrosternal thyroid – the trachea is often displaced and calci-fication is common

(c) aneurysm of the ascending aorta – may not calcify and aorto-graphy may be necessary for confirmation

(d) lymphoma – leukaemia is the commonest cause of an anterior mediastinal mass in a child, but calcification is rare.

Discussion

The mediastinum is divided into 4 major areas on the lateral chest radiograph.

(i) Superior mediastinum – the area above a line drawn from the upper end of the sternum to the 5th thoracic vertebra. The commonest mass is a retrosternal goitre. Vascular lesions are also important and arise from the subclavian or innominate arteries.

(ii) Anterior mediastinum – area anterior to the heart. Masses found here include retrosternal goitre, dermoids, teratomas, thymomas, pericardial cysts, diaphragmatic herniae, leukaemic or lymphomatous deposits and aneurysms of the ascending aorta.

(iii) Posterior mediastinum – extends from the posterior aspect of the heart to the vertebrae. Masses found in this region are neurogenic tumours, paravertebral abscesses, oesophageal lesions and aortic aneurysms.

(iv) Middle mediastinum – region occupied by the heart, great vessels and major bronchi. Masses in this region are likely to be bronchial carcinoma, lymphoma, sarcoidosis, primary tuberculosis and broncho-genic cysts.

Reference

Flower, C. D. R. (1976). Mediastinal Masses. *Hospital Update*, **2**, 295.

A50

Answers:

(1) Fusion of the sacro-iliac joints; para-spinal ligamentous ossification giving the appearance of 'bamboo spine'; relatively normal hip joints – this feature is important in assessing the prognosis for mobility. These features are characteristic of ankylosing spondylitis.

N.B., there is a left renal calculus.

(2) Acute leukaemia. In the late 1940s and early 1950s the treatment of ankylosing spondylitis was by large field application of X-rays to the spine and joints giving a dose of 12 000 rads or more. These patients are at least 5 times as likely as the control population to develop leukaemia, which may be chronic or acute myeloid leukaemia. The majority of patients present with leukaemia within 10 years of irradiation, but some present much later.

Section 3
DATA INTERPRETATION

AIDS FOR INTERPRETATION OF CARDIAC CATHETER DATA

Normal Pressures (mmHg)

Right atrium - mean 0-8

Right ventricle - less than 30/8 (= systolic/end-diastolic)

Pulmonary artery - less than 30/12 (mean 9-16)

Pulmonary artery wedge pressure (= left atrial pressure) 'a' wave less than 15, mean less than 10

Left ventricle - less than 140/12 (systolic pressure depends on systemic systolic blood pressure)

Abnormal Pressures

(1) Raised right ventricular systolic pressure due to pulmonary hypertension, pulmonary stenosis, Eisenmenger syndrome.

(2) Raised right ventricular end-diastolic pressure due to right ventricular failure, constrictive pericarditis, cardiomyopathy.

(3) Raised mean pulmonary artery pressure due to pulmonary hypertension, left to right shunt, mitral stenosis, left ventricular failure.

(4) Decreased mean pulmonary artery pressure due to pulmonary stenosis. (There must be a gradient greater than 20 mmHg before stenosis is diagnosed.)

(5) Raised pulmonary capillary wedge pressure due to mitral stenosis, mitral incompetence, left ventricular failure, aortic stenosis.

(6) Raised left ventricular systolic pressure due to systemic hypertension, aortic stenosis and non-valvular aortic stenosis including hypertrophic obstructive cardiomyopathy.

(7) Raised left ventricular end-diastolic pressure due to left ventricular failure, aortic incompetence, cardiomyopathy.

Diagnosis of Common Valve Lesions

(1) In aortic stenosis there is a pressure gradient between the left ventricular systolic pressure and the aortic systolic pressure.

(2) In aortic incompetence there is a wide pulse pressure and near equalization of the aortic and left ventricular end diastolic pressures.

(3) In mitral stenosis there is a difference between the pulmonary capillary wedge pressure (left atrial pressure) and the left ventricular diastolic pressure which is increased by exercise.

(4) If the right ventricular systolic pressure is equal to the aortic systolic pressure the diagnosis may be Eisenmenger syndrome, Fallot's tetralogy or transposition of the great vessels.

Shunts

In traditional oximetry multiple samples are taken in rapid succession from the following sites. Normal values for oxygen saturation are given.

Pulmonary artery (main left and right)	75%
Right ventricle (outflow, body, inflow)	75%
Right atrium (low, mid, high)	75%
Superior vena cava (low, high)	70%
Inferior vena cava at the level of diaphragm	80%
Brachial artery	95% +

If there is a left-to-right shunt the pulmonary blood flow is greater than the systemic blood flow. The position of oxygen step-up indicates the position of the shunt (for example in patent ductus arteriosis the step-up in oxygen saturation occurs between the right ventricle and the pulmonary artery).

If the shunt is from right to left there is arterial desaturation and the position of the shunt is indicated by the left heart chamber which is the first to show desaturation.

If the shunt is uni-directional its magnitude may be calculated as the difference between the pulmonary and systemic blood flows. This can be simply calculated approximately using the formula – (systemic arterial oxygen saturation minus mixed venous oxygen saturation) divided by (systemic arterial oxygen saturation minus pulmonary artery oxygen saturation).

An accepted formula for calculating the mixed venous oxygen saturation is:

$$3 \times \text{SVC oxygen saturation} + 1 \times \text{IVC oxygen saturation} \div 4$$

Q1 A 39-year-old man presents with dizzy spells, weight loss and glycosuria. He has a standard 75 g oral glucose tolerance test, the results of which are shown in the following table:

Time (min)	Blood Glucose (mmol/l)	Urine Glucose
0	5	0
30	13.5	+ +
60	6	+
90	2.1	0
120	5.1	0

Questions:
(1) What is your interpretation of this glucose tolerance test?
(2) What are the causes of the abnormality?

Q2 A 20-year-old man having chemotherapy for acute myeloid leukaemia is given a blood transfusion to correct his anaemia. He is then noted to be breathless and his lung function tests and arterial blood gases are as follows:

Vital capacity	4.7 litres (predicted 5.5 l)
FEV$_1$	3.6 l (predicted 4.2 l)
P_aCO_2	3.8 kPa
P_aO_2	8.5 kPa
DLco (carbon monoxide transfer factor single breath)	28 ml/min/mmHg (predicted 17 ml/min/mmHg)

Questions:
(1) Comment on these results.
(2) Suggest the most likely cause of the abnormalities.

Questions:

Q3

Two samples of blood have been taken within 10 minutes of each other from the same vein of a patient. What is the most likely explanation of the difference between the 2 samples?

	Sample 1	Sample 2
Haemoglobin	13.6 g/dl	14.3 g/dl
Plasma potassium	4.2 mmol/l	4.1 mmol/l
Serum calcium	2.3 mmol/l	2.51 mmol/l
Serum albumin	41 g/l	45 g/l
Serum thyroxine	96 nmol/l	107 nmol/l

A 47-year-old man presents with recurrent painless jaundice. Investigations show:

Q4

Haemoglobin 9.2 g/dl
MCV 117 fl
White cell count $2.3 \times 10^9/l$
Platelets $90 \times 10^9/l$
Reticulocytes 7%
Serum bilirubin 95 μmol/l
Alkaline phosphatase 130 U/l
SGPT 35 U/l
Antinuclear factor negative
Direct Antiglobulin (Coombs) test negative

The patient's red cells show lysis in the presence of acid and normal serum but no lysis in acidified heat inactivated serum.

Questions:

(1) What is the diagnosis?
(2) What are the causes of death associated with this condition?

Q5 The following results were obtained by Cardiac Catheterization:

	Pressure (mmHg)	Oxygen saturation (%)
Superior vena cava	mean 4	74
Inferior vena cava	mean 2	68
High right atrium		75
Mid right atrium	mean 4	74
Low right atrium		76
Right ventricle body	40/0 end-diastole 3	81
Right ventricle outflow tract	40/0	88
Pulmonary artery	40/15 mean 24	88
Left ventricle	110/2 end-diastole 7	99

Questions:
(1) Comment on these results.
(2) Suggest the likely diagnosis.

Q6 The following thyroid function tests are from a woman with dysthyroid eye disease.

Serum thyroxine 95 nmol/l
Serum triiodothyronine 2.1 nmol/l

TRH. test (200 µg thyrotrophin given intravenously at time 0 minutes):

0 minutes	TSH 4 mU/l
20 minutes	TSH 6 mU/l
60 minutes	TSH 5 mU/l

Questions:
(1) Comment on these results.
(2) Give 3 possible explanations for the abnormality.
(3) What further investigations would you suggest?

A 66-year-old woman with severe Raynaud's phenomenon complains of dysphagia and a recurrent dry cough associated with fever. Biochemical investigations reveal the following:

Q7

Serum albumin	35 g/l
Serum globulins	40 g/l
IgA	3.0 g/l
IgG	10 g/l
IgM	8.2 g/l
Alkaline phosphatase	1250 U/l
SGPT	35 U/l
Serum bilirubin	21 μmol/l

Questions:
(1) Give 2 likely diagnoses.
(2) What other investigation would you perform to support these diagnoses?
(3) How may the recurrent cough be explained?

A 26-year-old, three weeks postpartum, is admitted because of bruising and epistaxis. There is no past history of bleeding disorder and the delivery was uneventful. The following laboratory investigations were performed:

Q8

Haemoglobin 11 g/dl
White cell count 13.2 × 10⁹/l
Platelet count 150 × 10⁹/l
Hess test negative
Kaolin partial thromboplastin time (KPTT) 72 s (control 40 s)
Prothrombin time 13 s (control 14 s)
Plasma fibrinogen 3.7 g/l (normal 1.5–3.5)

Questions:
(1) What further investigations would be useful?
(2) Give possible causes to explain these haematological abnormalities.

Q9

A 13-year-old boy presents with a 1-year history of increasing shortness of breath on exertion. Cardiac catheterization is performed and the following results obtained:

	Pressure (mmHg)	Oxygen saturation (%)
Superior vena cava		66
Inferior vena cava		78
High right atrium	2 (mean)	86
Mid right atrium		94
Low right atrium		80
Right ventricle	60/0	87
Pulmonary artery	16/8 (10 mean)	87
Femoral artery		96

Questions:
(1) Give 2 diagnoses.
(2) What other information can be derived from these figures?

Q10

The table shows 2 sets of results performed on the same sample of plasma taken from an acutely ill patient.

	A		B	
Sodium	101	(mmol/l)	131	(mmol/l)
Potassium	3.5	,,	4.8	,,
Bicarbonate	11	,,	14	,,
Glucose	21.3	,,	28.8	,,
Urea	3.9	,,	6.4	,,
Creatinine '	106	(μmol/l)	138	(μmol/l)

Questions:
(1) What procedure has been performed to give the values B?
(2) What is the diagnosis in this patient?
(3) How do you account for the differences in the values in columns A and B?

A 35-year-old lady was found to be hypertensive, hypokalaemic and had noted a recent increase in weight. She was admitted for a dexamethasone suppression test, and the following results were obtained:

9 am plasma cortisol 900 nmol/l (normal range 170–720 nmol/l)

Following 0.5 mg of dexamethasone 6-hourly for 48 hours, 9 am plasma cortisol 600 nmol/l

Dexamethasone 2 mg 6-hourly for 48 hours reduced the 9 am plasma cortisol to 150 nmol/l.

Q11

Questions:
(1) Suggest a likely diagnosis.
(2) Comment on the specificity of this test.
(3) What further investigation may help to confirm your diagnosis?

A 59-year-old woman had the following blood count:

Q12

    Haemoglobin 20.1 g/dl

    PCV 68%

    MCV 83 fl

    MCHC 31 g/dl

    White cell count 9.0×10^9/l (normal differential)

    Platelets 220×10^9/l

    Arterial blood gases:

      Po_2 11 kPa

      Pco_2 5 kPa

    Electrolytes, urea and creatinine normal

Questions:
Give 4 possible causes for these results.

Q13

A 79-year-old lady is admitted with diarrhoea and vomiting. Oral fluid replacement is encouraged. You are called to see her 24 h later because she has passed only 350 ml of urine.

Questions
(1) Comment on the following results:
   plasma sodium 129 mmol/l, potassium 3.1 mmol/l, urea 20 mmol/l, creatinine 215 μmol/l, glucose 7 mmol/l
   urinary sodium 15 mmol/l, urea 300 mmol/l, osmolarity 640 mosmol/l
(2) What management would be appropriate?

Q14

You receive the following report about a patient seen the previous evening. The venepuncture was difficult and a small needle was used.
   Plasma sodium 136 mmol/l, potassium 8.9 mmol/l, urea 14.6 mmol/l, bicarbonate 19 mmol/l, creatinine 220 μmol/l, glucose 1.8 mmol/l
   Serum calcium 2.1 mmol/l, phosphate 3.8 mmol/l

Questions:
How would you explain these results?

Q15

In the investigation of a patient with renal stones, raised ESR and possible hyperparathyroidism an uncuffed, fasting venous sample gave the following results:
   Plasma sodium 136 mmol/l, potassium 8.2 mmol/l, urea 7.8 mmol/l, bicarbonate 29 mmol/l
   Serum calcium 0.9 mmol/l, phosphate 1.2 mmol/l

Questions:
Explain these results.

A 27-year-old man with a past history of self-poisoning is found unconscious and hyperventilating. His breath does not smell of alcohol. Biochemical investigations are as follows:

Plasma sodium 154 mmol/l, potassium 4.8 mmol/l, chloride 91 mmol/l, bicarbonate 5 mmol/l, urea 9.0 mmol/l, creatinine 120 μmol/l, glucose 9.0 mmol/l

Q16

Questions:
Give 4 useful tests to determine the cause of his coma.

Questions:
Give 3 possible causes for these cerebro-spinal fluid findings:

glucose 4.2 mmol/l (simultaneous plasma glucose 5.8 mmol/l)
protein 4.7 g/l
cells – 3 lymphocytes per mm^3
culture sterile

Q17

You are asked to see a patient with acute abdominal pain who has been admitted for emergency surgery. The anaesthetist is worried about the patient's diabetes because of the following results on a venous blood sample:

Plasma sodium 123 mmol/l, potassium 2.9 mmol/l, urea 4.0 mmol/l, glucose 43 mmol/l, bicarbonate 19 mmol/l

Q18

Questions:
What would you advise?

Q19

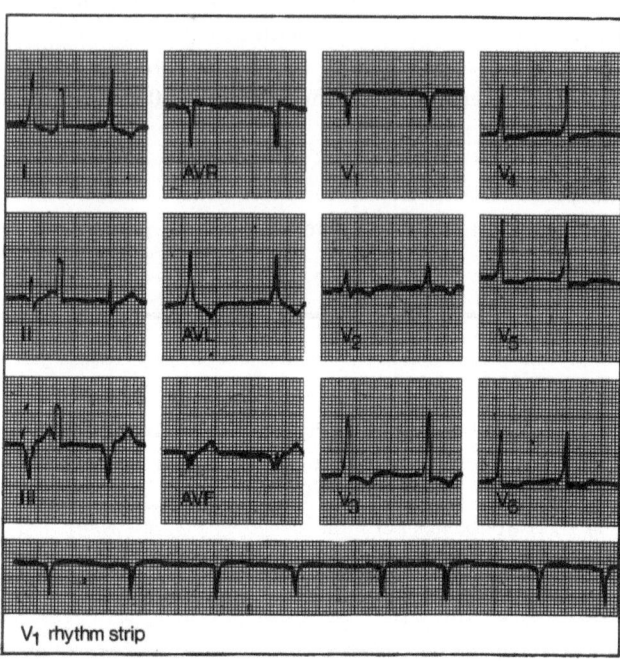

V₁ rhythm strip

Questions:

(1) Document the abnormalities shown on this electrocardiogram.

(2) What is the diagnosis?

(3) How may the patient have presented?

Q20

The shaded areas on the diagram facing are the visual fields (plotted with a Hamblin perimeter) of a 40-year-old man whose presenting complaint was of headaches.

Questions:

(1) Describe the abnormality.

(2) Discuss possible causes.

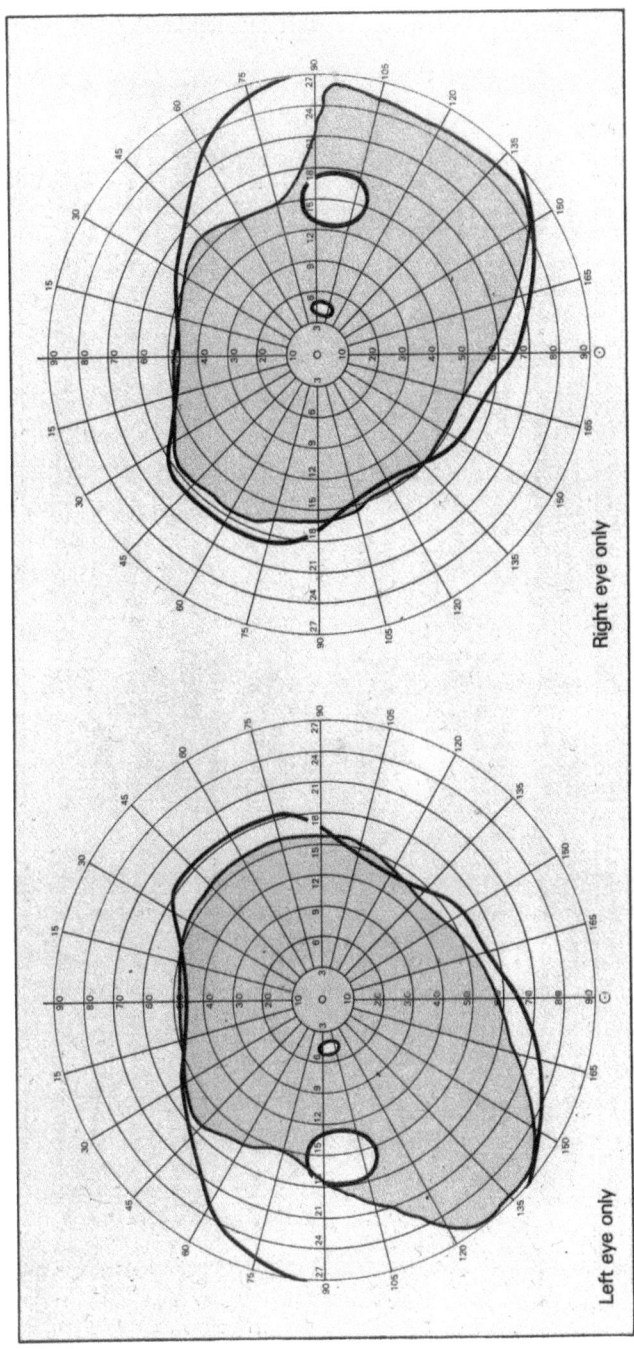

Q21

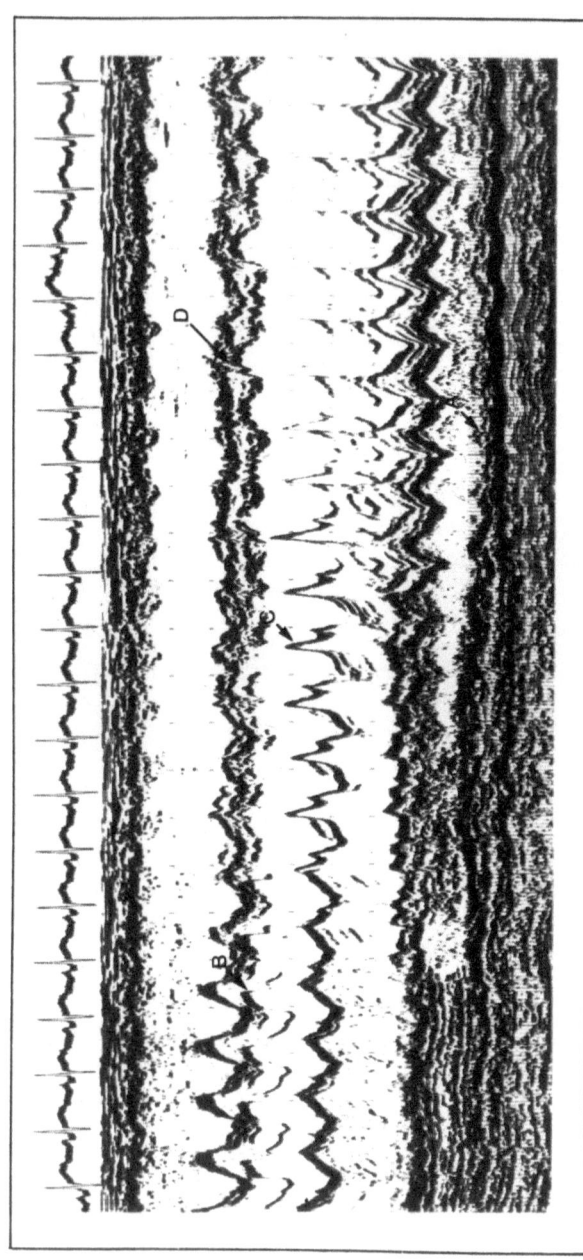

This echocardiogram was recorded from a 26-year-old man who presented with central chest pain, fever and breathlessness, associated with an influenza-like illness.

Questions:
(1) What are the structures labelled A, B, C and D?
(2) What abnormality does the echocardiogram show?
(3) What is the likely diagnosis?

Answers:

A1

(1) The peak blood glucose level is abnormally high, but the fasting and 2 hour values are within normal limits. Blood glucose falls to a hypoglycaemic level at 90 minutes. This is a lag-storage curve.

(2) The lag-storage curve occurs:
   (a) in apparently normal individuals with reactive hypoglycaemia.
   (b) after gastrectomy, when rapid entry of carbohydrate into the intestine leads to rapid absorption (late dumping syndrome).
   (c) in severe liver disease due to abnormal glycogen metabolism.
   (d) in hyperthyroidism.
   (e) as an early manifestation of diabetes mellitus.

This patient's dizzy spells may be due to hypoglycaemia. His weight loss may be due to hyperthyroidism or may be the result of a previous partial gastrectomy. Glycosuria is a manifestation of the lag-storage.

Answers:

A2

(1) Lung function tests show a mild restrictive ventilatory defect with no obstructive element. The arterial blood gases show hypoxaemia (low P_aO_2) with evidence of hyperventilation (low P_aCO_2). The transfer factor is markedly elevated which is characteristic of intra-alveolar haemorrhage.

(2) The most likely diagnosis is lung haemorrhage secondary to thrombocytopenia. Anaemia will tend to lower the transfer factor towards normal, but in this patient the anaemia has been corrected by blood transfusion.

Other causes of an elevated transfer factor (usually not as marked as this) include asthma and pulmonary oedema which would be a possible diagnosis in this patient following his blood transfusion.

A3

Answers:
The difference between the 2 samples can be explained by the first sample having been taken with the patient in the recumbent position, and the second in the upright position following 10 minutes ambulation. When standing, elevated dependent venous pressure causes small molecules and water to pass into the tissue space leading to an increased concentration of protein, haemoglobin and protein bound molecules. The serum albumin may be between 5 and 10 g/l higher in the upright position compared to the recumbent.

A similar discrepancy between 2 blood samples could occur following prolonged venous stasis at the site of venepuncture. In this situation the plasma potassium would be elevated because of local hypoxia. The resulting acidosis causes a leak of potassium from the cells into the plasma.

A4

Answers:
(1) There is pancytopenia with evidence of haemolysis (raised bilirubin, macrocytosis and reticulocytosis). It is unlikely that the haemolysis is due to a serum antibody as the direct antiglobulin test and antinuclear factor are negative. There is no lysis of red cells in the absence of complement (heat inactivated serum) and this makes it unlikely that spherocytosis is present. The cells are abnormally susceptible to lysis by complement (provided by normal serum) in the presence of acid. This is Ham's test and the result suggests paroxysmal nocturnal haemoglobinuria. There is also pancytopenia which is consistent with this diagnosis.

(2) The causes of death associated with this condition are:
   (a) aplastic anaemia
   (b) venous thromboses, particularly of the portal system and brain
   (c) infection due to leucopenia and defective leucocyte function
   (d) paroxysmal nocturnal haemoglobinuria which may rarely progress to leukaemia.

Answers:

A5

(1) (a) There is a step-up in oxygen saturation between the right atrium and the body of the right ventricle with a further increase in the right ventricular out-flow tract. This suggests a left-to-right shunt at ventricular level.

(b) The right ventricular systolic pressure is elevated (normally less than 30/8 mmHg) in keeping with the presence of a left-to-right shunt at ventricular level.

(2) Ventricular septal defect with left-to-right shunt.

The pulmonary:systemic blood flow ratio is approximately 2:1.

Answers:

A6

(1) The serum T4 and T3 are both within normal limits. The basal TSH is normal but there is no significant response of TSH to the injected TRH. This is a 'flat' TRH test.

(2) An absent TSH response to injected TRH suggests that thyroid hormone secretion is slightly excessive or that thyroid function is autonomous. A normal response, however, excludes the diagnosis of thyrotoxicosis.

(a) Graves's disease (either euthyroid or hyperthyroid)

(b) Multinodular goitre

(c) Old age (particularly males)

(d) Steroid therapy

N.B. Pituitary failure is unlikely because the T4 is normal.

(3) The normal T4 and T3 make hyperthyroidism unlikely unless these values are spurious due to alterations in binding proteins. Further investigations would include measurement of thyroid binding globulins, free thyroxine index and measurement of free thyroxine.

A7

Answers:

(1) Primary biliary cirrhosis and systemic sclerosis.

These 2 conditions may be associated. The diagnosis of primary biliary cirrhosis is suggested by an elevation of serum IgM and alkaline phosphatase, and of systemic sclerosis by the combination of dysphagia (from oesophageal involvement) and Raynaud's phenomenon.

(2) Tests that help to confirm the diagnosis of primary biliary cirrhosis are:

   (a) gamma-glutamyl transpeptidase/5-nucleotidase estimations, or determination of alkaline phosphatase iso-enzymes to confirm that the elevated alkaline phosphatase is hepatic in origin. A greatly elevated alkaline phosphatase in the absence of biochemical evidence of abnormal liver function suggests Paget's disease of bone, metastatic liver disease or primary biliary cirrhosis.

   (b) anti-mitochondrial antibodies. These are present in over 95% of patients with primary biliary cirrhosis, and when in high titre are specific for this disorder.

   (c) percutaneous liver biopsy.

The diagnosis of systemic sclerosis is made primarily on clinical grounds. The following may be helpful:

   (a) X-ray of hands to demonstrate subcutaneous calcinosis.

   (b) Barium swallow to demonstrate decreased oesophageal peristalsis.

   (c) Positive antinuclear antibodies with negative DNA binding. This, and other auto-antibody tests are non-specific.

(3) Repeated aspiration pneumonia from the dilated stagnant oesophagus.

A8

Answers:

(1) (a) Repeat the kaolin partial thromboplastin time (KPTT) after the addition of normal plasma to see if the abnormality is corrected. If uncorrected, this suggests circulating inhibitors of clotting.

   (b) Factor VIII assay

(c) Factor IX assay

(d) Antinuclear antibody

(2) KPTT measures the factors involved in the intrinsic pathway of the clotting mechanism (Factors XII, XI, X, IX, VIII and V). The test measures the time in which plasma, previously incubated with kaolin, takes to clot in the presence of an optimum amount of platelet lipid substitute and calcium. Kaolin provides the maximum stimulus for activation of Factor XII, and cephalin (an ether extract of human brain) is a platelet substitute. When the KPTT is prolonged and the prothrombin time is normal (this measures Factors VII, X, V, prothrombin and fibrinogen) there is usually a deficiency of either Factor VIII or IX or inhibitors of Factor VIII. (There may also be deficiency of Factors XII and XI, but this is unusual.)

The disorders associated with defects of the intrinsic pathway are:

(a) Haemophilia as a result of deficiency or abnormality of Factor VIII, Factor IX or von Willebrand's disease.

(b) Acquired circulating inhibitors of coagulation, usually directed against Factor VIII, associated with:

(i) pregnancy. The abnormality occurs within the first few weeks to several months after delivery and usually disappears spontaneously.

(ii) systemic lupus erythematosus. Various inhibitors are described, including anti-Factor VIII.

(iii) rheumatoid arthritis.

(iv) carcinoma.

(v) lymphoma.

(vi) pemphigus.

(vii) dermatitis herpetiformis.

(viii) normal elderly subjects.

Where there is a major bleeding diathesis, the treatment is immunosuppressive therapy with cyclophosphamide or azathioprine and steroids. Factor VIII concentrates should not be used alone as they may boost antibody titres and should be reserved for life-threatening haemorrhage.

A9

Answers:

(1) (a) Atrial septal defect (ASD)

    (b) Pulmonary stenosis

Oximetry shows an abnormal step-up in saturation at the level of the mid right atrium, typical of a secundum ASD. The right ventricular systolic pressure is high compared with the pulmonary artery pressure, suggestive of out-flow tract obstruction.

(2) (a) The peak systolic right ventricular out-flow tract gradient is 44 mmHg

    (b) The pulmonary: systemic blood flow ratio is 3 : 1.

A10

Answers:

(1) Ether extraction of lipid

(2) Diabetes mellitus with associated hyperlipidaemia

(3) This is pseudo-hyponatraemia which may occur in the presence of severe hyperlipidaemia or hyperproteinaemia. Sodium ions are distributed in the aqueous phase of plasma, and in the above conditions the volume of distribution is much lower than the volume of the sample. Measured sodium is expressed as if it were present in the total volume and is therefore reported as low.

A11

Answers:

(1) Cushing's disease (pituitary-dependent bilateral adrenal hyperplasia).

(2) Failure of suppression of morning plasma cortisol on a low dose (2 mg daily) of dexamethasone suggests a diagnosis of Cushing's syndrome (hypercorticolism), although this is sometimes seen in obesity, depression and in some hospital patients, particularly if stressed. Suppression by high dose (8 mg daily) of dexamethasone indicates Cushing's disease (pituitary-dependent bilateral adrenal hyperplasia). Patients with ectopic ACTH production, adrenal adenoma or carcinoma usually do not suppress, even with high

dose dexamethasone. There are, however, exceptions to this rule, including some patients with depression and pseudo-Cushing's syndrome (enzyme induction seen in alcoholics) who may not suppress even on high dose. In this latter case the diagnosis is usually made by reduction in hypercorticalism following admission to hospital (and consequent abstinence from alcohol). The results of dexamethasone suppression should therefore not be taken in isolation in the investigation of patients with apparent hypersecretion of cortisol.

(3) The useful confirmatory test to establish the diagnosis of Cushing's disease is the plasma ACTH level. This will be completely suppressed if there is a primary adrenal disorder; it will be elevated with pituitary dependent Cushing's disease and will be very high in the presence of ectopic ACTH production (although there is some overlap).

Answers:

A12

There is polycythaemia with a normal number of white cells and platelets. This makes the diagnosis of polycythaemia rubra vera unlikely. The blood gases exclude hypoxia causing secondary polycythaemia. The most likely diagnosis therefore is over production of erythropoietin as a result of

(a) kidney tumour
(b) carcinoma of the liver
(c) cerebellar haemangioblastoma
(d) uterine myomata
(e) phaeochromocytoma
(f) virilizing syndrome.

Measurement of red cell mass and plasma volume should confirm true polycythaemia and help to exclude Gaisböck's syndrome (low plasma volume seen in men who smoke). The normal electrolytes, urea and creatinine make dehydration very unlikely as a cause of the raised haemoglobin.

A13 Answers:

(1) The plasma urea is raised relatively more than the creatinine which suggests dehydration. The urine–plasma urea ratio is 15:1 (greater than 10:1 suggesting pre-renal failure as the cause of oliguria). The low urinary sodium (less than 20 mmol/l) also suggests appropriate response to dehydration. The calculated plasma osmolarity is 291 mosmol/l giving a urine–plasma osmolar ratio greater than 1.8:1, in keeping with pre-renal oliguria.

(2) The management should be intravenous rehydration with saline, and potassium replacement.

A14 Answers:

The blood sample was analysed on the morning after being taken and the whole blood was allowed to stand overnight prior to separation of the cells from the plasma. During this time intracellular molecules can leak into the plasma (potassium and phosphate) and red cells continue to metabolize glucose accounting for the low plasma glucose (unless the sample has been put into a bottle containing fluoride which specifically inhibits glucose metabolism). A similar picture may be seen if the sample is haemolysed but in this situation the plasma glucose will not be low.

A15 Answers:

A difficult venepuncture failed to yield enough blood for haematological and biochemical investigations. Some blood from the sequestrene bottle (haematology) was added to the lithium heparin (biochemistry) bottle. Sequesterene (EDTA) acts as an anti-coagulant by binding calcium, and the potassium salt is usually used. The raised potassium and low calcium in this sample can be explained in this way. A raised potassium cannot be explained on the basis of haemolysis as this does not explain the low calcium, and the phosphate would be high in this circumstance.

Answers:

A16

(1) A test for the presence of ketones in the urine (either diabetic or alcoholic ketosis). Remember that Acetest and Ketostix respond only to aceto-acetic acid and a significant keto-acidosis may be present with the excretion of only beta-hydroxybutyrate (particularly in states of low oxygenation). The blood glucose is not necessarily markedly elevated in diabetic keto-acidosis.

(2) Plasma lactate. Acidosis in the absence of ketonuria suggests lactic acidosis. This is associated with an anion gap of greater than 20 mmol/l.

(3) Plasma salicylate level – rare to cause such severe acidosis in adults, but will produce hyperventilation. The urine may be tested with a 10% solution of ferric chloride which gives a red colour in the presence of salicylate (the urine should be boiled to destroy aceto-acetic acid which gives a similar reaction).

(4) Plasma osmolarity – the calculated osmolarity $[2 \times (Na + K) + urea + glucose]$ is 330 mosmol/l. The measured osmolarity in this case was 420 mosmol/l. Ethanol, methanol and ethylene glycol will increase osmolarity, the latter two causing symptoms of alcohol poisoning without the characteristic smell.

(5) Renal tubular acidosis (remember acetazolamide) should be considered but the plasma potassium is usually low and the chloride high.

Answers:

A17

The protein is markedly raised in the absence of an increase in cells. The following explanations would be compatible with these results:

(1) post-infective polyneuropathy (Guillain–Barré syndrome).
   In this condition the CSF usually contains few cells and the pressure is normal. In 10% of patients there may be up to 50 cells per mm³, predominantly lymphocytes. The protein concentration may be normal early in the disease.

(2) CNS tumours, particularly acoustic neuroma.

(3) spinal block (Froin's syndrome).

A18

Answers:

It is unlikely that the elevated blood glucose could be explained by a hyperosmolar non-ketotic diabetic state, as this is usually associated with dehydration and the plasma urea and sodium would be elevated. Diabetic ketoacidosis would also be associated with dehydration and a lower plasma bicarbonate. The likely explanation for these results is that the blood sample has been taken proximal to an intravenous infusion of dextrose. The advice would be to change the infusion to physiological saline (particularly if the patient has been vomiting in association with the acute abdominal emergency). The venepuncture should be repeated on the arm which does not have the intravenous infusion.

A19

(1) P–R interval of less than 0.10 seconds; wide QRS complex; slurred onset of the upstroke of the R wave – the delta wave; QS in lead III and AVF; T wave invertion in leads I, AVL, V2 and V3; flat T waves in V4 to V6.

(2) Wolff–Parkinson–White Syndrome Type B (negative delta and QS in V1). The abnormalities in lead III and AVF suggest inferior myocardial infarction, but this electrocardiographic diagnosis should be avoided in the presence of pre-excitation.

(3) This syndrome may present:
    (a) incidentally as an electrocardiographic diagnosis
    (b) as paroxysmal tachycardia
    (c) with a family history of tachycardia
    (d) with associated congenital heart disease, particularly abnormalities of the tricuspid valve.

Answers:

(1) An incongruous bitemporal hemianopia.

A20

(2) Chiasmal compression with bitemporal field defects is the characteristic finding in patients with pituitary tumours and suprasellar extension.

Similar defects may also be seen with
   (a) parasellar tumours
   (b) vascular abnormalities
   (c) plaques of demyelination at the chiasma
   (d) focal retinitis pigmentosa
   (e) following irradiation to the chiasma
   (f) cerebral sarcoidosis

It should be noted that the field defects associated with pituitary tumours may be asymmetrical, and usually start with an upper quadrantinopia.

Answers:

(1) (A) Parietal pericardium.
    (B) Aortic valve.
    (C) Anterior leaflet of the mitral valve.
    (D) Interventricular septum.

A21

(2) Posterior pericardial effusion.

(3) Acute pericarditis.

This echocardiogram is a slow scan from the aorta to the left ventricle. Note that the anterior wall of the aorta is continuous with the interventricular septum, and the posterior wall with the anterior leaflet of the mitral valve. The left atrium lies behind the aorta and the interventricular septum divides the right ventricle from the left ventricle. There is an echo-free space behind the posterior wall of the left ventricle (between the dense lines of the parietal and epicardial pericardium), and this indicates the presence of a pericardial effusion. Characteristically, the effusion disappears as the transducer scans from the left ventricle to the aorta.

The echocardiogram is the most sensitive method of detecting a pericardial effusion. The patient's history suggests that the effusion is associated with viral pericarditis.

At the time of going to press an echocardiogram had not been included in the MRCP Examination Data Interpretation. It is, however, becoming an increasingly valuable investigation in patients with general medical conditions, and candidates should be aware of its applications and basic interpretation.

INDEX

179